The Long Goodbye: Caring for Loved Ones Through End-of-Life Care

By
Cynthia Kemlage
LVN, SWOC, CDP, C.A.L.M, Death Doula

Disclaimer

The information contained in this book is for informational and educational purposes only and is not intended as a substitute for professional medical advice, diagnosis, or treatment. It is essential to consult with qualified healthcare professionals, such as physicians, nurses, and other relevant specialists, for any questions or concerns you may have regarding end-of-life care, medical conditions, treatment options, or specific healthcare decisions. The information presented in this book should not be used to make medical decisions on your own or on behalf of another person.

End-of-life care is a complex and highly individualized process. The recommendations, suggestions, and examples provided in this book are general in nature and may not be applicable to every situation. Each person's circumstances, medical history, and personal preferences are unique, and it is crucial to work closely with your healthcare team to develop a personalized care plan that meets your specific needs.

This book does not endorse or recommend any specific treatments, medications, healthcare providers, or facilities. The mention of any specific organization, website, or individual does not constitute an endorsement. It is your responsibility to research and choose healthcare providers, treatments, and facilities that are appropriate for your individual needs and circumstances.

Table of Contents

Part 4
Supporting the Caregiver

Part 5
Practical Considerations and Resources

Part 1

Understanding End-of-Life Care

Chapter 1

Defining End-of-Life Care

The journey of caring for a loved one nearing the end of their life is a deeply personal and often challenging experience. It's a time filled with complex emotions, difficult decisions, and the profound desire to provide comfort and support during this final chapter. Before we delve into the practicalities and emotional nuances of end-of-life care, it's important to establish a clear understanding of what it encompasses and, perhaps even more importantly, what it *doesn't* mean.

End-of-life Care is not About Giving Up

It's not about hastening death. Instead, it's a specialized approach to healthcare that focuses on providing comfort, dignity, and support to individuals and their families facing a life-limiting illness. It shifts the focus from curative treatments aimed at prolonging life to maximizing the quality of remaining life. This shift often involves a re-evaluation of priorities, where comfort and peace become paramount.

It's important to understand that "end-of-life" doesn't necessarily refer to the final days or hours. It can encompass a period of months, or even years, during which an individual is living with a terminal illness or facing a significant decline in health. This period can be marked by varying degrees of physical and emotional challenges, and end-of-life care adapts to meet these evolving needs.

One of the most significant distinctions in end-of-life care is the transition from curative to palliative care. Curative care focuses on treating the underlying disease and attempting to achieve a cure. Palliative care, on the other hand, focuses on relieving pain and other symptoms, regardless of the stage of the illness. While palliative care can be integrated alongside curative treatment, at a certain point, the emphasis shifts entirely to palliative care as the focus becomes solely on comfort and quality of life. This transition can be difficult to navigate, both for the individual and their family, and it often requires open and honest conversations with the healthcare team. Several factors contribute to the complexity of defining end-of-life care:

- **Individualized Experiences:** Every individual's experience of dying is unique. There is no single "right" way to approach end-of-life care, and the needs and preferences of each person must be respected.

- **Varying Trajectories:** The course of a terminal illness can be unpredictable. Some individuals may experience a gradual decline, while others may have a more erratic trajectory with periods of relative stability followed by rapid deterioration.

- **Emotional and Spiritual Needs:** End-of-life care addresses not only the physical needs of the individual but also their emotional and spiritual well-being. This includes addressing fears, anxieties, and unresolved issues, as well as providing opportunities for meaning-making and connection.

- **Family Involvement:** End-of-life care recognizes the importance of family involvement. It aims to support the entire family unit, providing education, emotional support, and bereavement care.

The Philosophy of End-of-Life Care: Shifting Focus from Cure to Comfort

End-of-life care represents a profound shift in the healthcare paradigm, moving away from a primary focus on curing disease to prioritizing comfort, dignity, and quality of life in the face of a life-limiting illness. This philosophical shift is not about abandoning hope but rather redefining it. It acknowledges the reality of mortality and seeks to support individuals and their families through the final stages of life with compassion and respect.

The Limitations of Cure

Modern medicine has made remarkable strides in treating and curing diseases. However, there comes a point in some illnesses where curative treatments may no longer be effective, or their side effects may outweigh their benefits. Continuing aggressive treatments in these situations can sometimes prolong suffering rather than extend meaningful life.

Recognizing these limitations is a crucial step in embracing the philosophy of end-of-life care.

Redefining Hope

In end-of-life care, hope doesn't disappear; it evolves. The focus shifts from hoping for a cure to hoping for:

- **Comfort:** Freedom from pain and other distressing symptoms.

- **Connection:** Meaningful time with loved ones and the opportunity to express love and gratitude.

- **Dignity:** Maintaining a sense of self and control throughout the dying process.

- **Peace:** A sense of closure, acceptance, and spiritual well-being.

- **Quality of Life:** Making the most of the time remaining, however limited it may be.

The Core Principles of End-of-Life Care

The philosophy of end-of-life care is grounded in several core principles:

- **Respect for Autonomy:** Individuals have the right to make decisions about their own care, including the right to refuse treatment. End-of-life care prioritizes respecting these choices and supporting individuals in exercising their autonomy.

- **Focus on the Person:** End-of-life care recognizes that individuals are more than their illness. It emphasizes treating the whole person – physical, emotional, social, and spiritual – and addressing their unique needs and concerns.

- **Symptom Management:** Controlling pain and other distressing symptoms is a central focus. The goal is to maximize comfort and minimize suffering, allowing individuals to live as fully as possible.

- **Emotional and Spiritual Support:** End-of-life care addresses the emotional and spiritual needs of both the individual and their family. This may involve counseling, support groups, spiritual guidance, and opportunities for meaning-making and reflection.

- **Family-Centered Care:** Families are an integral part of the end-of-life experience. End-of-life care supports families by providing education, emotional support, and bereavement services.

- **Quality over Quantity:** The emphasis shifts from prolonging life at all costs to maximizing the quality of remaining life. This may involve making difficult decisions about foregoing aggressive treatments in favor of comfort-focused care.

- **Dignity and Respect:** End-of-life care aims to preserve the individual's dignity and respect throughout the dying process. This includes honoring their wishes, respecting their privacy, and treating them with compassion and empathy.

The Role of the Healthcare Team

The healthcare team plays a vital role in providing end-of-life care. They work collaboratively with the individual and their family to:

- **Assess Needs:** Identify the individual's physical, emotional, social, and spiritual needs.

- **Develop a Care Plan:** Create a personalized care plan that addresses these needs and aligns with the individual's wishes.

- **Manage Symptoms:** Provide expert symptom management to maximize comfort.

- **Offer Support:** Provide emotional and spiritual support to both the individual and their family.

- **Facilitate Communication:** Facilitate open and honest communication about end-of-life issues.

The Benefits of End-of-Life Care

Embracing the philosophy of end-of-life care can have numerous benefits:

- **Improved Quality of Life:** Individuals can experience a better quality of life in their final stages, free from unnecessary suffering.

- **Enhanced Comfort:** Effective symptom management can significantly improve comfort and well-being.

- **Greater Emotional and Spiritual Well-being:** Addressing emotional and spiritual needs can lead to a greater sense of peace and closure.

- **Increased Family Satisfaction:** Families often report greater satisfaction with the care provided when the focus is on comfort and support.

- **Reduced Burden on Caregivers:** End-of-life care can provide support for caregivers, reducing their burden and improving their ability to provide care.

The philosophy of end-of-life care represents a compassionate and person-centered approach to caring for individuals facing a life-limiting illness. By shifting the focus from cure to comfort, it allows individuals to live their final stages of life with dignity, respect, and the best possible quality of life. It's about embracing a holistic approach that acknowledges the reality of mortality and supports individuals and their families through this profound and often transformative experience.

What End-of-Life Care Is and What It Isn't

What End-of-Life Care Is

- **Holistic Approach:** End-of-life care addresses the physical, emotional, social, and spiritual needs of the individual. It recognizes that dying is a multifaceted experience and aims to support the whole person.

- **Patient-Centered:** The individual's preferences, values, and wishes are at the heart of end-of-life care. The goal is to empower individuals to make choices that align with their personal goals and priorities.

- **Comfort-Focused:** A primary objective is to manage pain and other distressing symptoms to ensure the individual is as comfortable as possible. This includes both medical and non-medical approaches to symptom management.

- **Supportive:** End-of-life care provides support not only for the individual but also for their family and loved ones. This includes education, counseling, and bereavement support.

- **Adaptive:** End-of-life care is flexible and adapts to the changing needs of the individual as their illness progresses. It recognizes that the dying process is unique to each person and requires individualized care plans.

- **Dignified:** End-of-life care aims to preserve the individual's dignity and respect throughout the dying process. It emphasizes honoring their autonomy and ensuring they are treated with compassion and empathy.

What End-of-Life Care Isn't

- **Giving Up:** Choosing end-of-life care is not about giving up on life. It's about shifting the focus from curative treatments that may no longer be effective to maximizing the quality of remaining life.

- **Hastening Death:** End-of-life care does not hasten death. It focuses on providing comfort and support, allowing the natural dying process to unfold without intervention.

- **Only for the Final Days:** End-of-life care is not solely for the final days or hours of life. It can be appropriate for months or even years, depending on the individual's circumstances and the progression of their illness.

- **One-Size-Fits-All:** There is no single "right" way to approach end-of-life care. It is a highly individualized process that takes into account the unique needs and preferences of each person.

- **Just About Physical Needs:** While managing physical symptoms is a pivotal component, end-of-life care also addresses emotional, social, and spiritual needs. It recognizes that these aspects are equally important in ensuring a peaceful and meaningful end-of-life experience.

- **A Replacement for Curative Care:** In some cases, end-of-life care can be provided alongside curative treatment. The transition to end-of-life care often occurs gradually as the focus shifts from cure to comfort.

Key Considerations

- **Communication:** Open and honest communication is essential in end-of-life care. This includes discussions about goals of care, advance directives, and end-of-life wishes.

- **Advance Care Planning:** It's important for individuals to engage in advance care planning to make their wishes known regarding future medical care. This may involve creating a living will or designating a durable power of attorney for healthcare.

- **Family Involvement:** End-of-life care recognizes the importance of family involvement. It aims to support the entire family unit, providing education, emotional support, and bereavement care.

Debunking Common Myths

Unfortunately, several misconceptions surround end-of-life care, which can create unnecessary fear and anxiety. It's important to debunk these myths to foster a more informed and compassionate understanding:

- **Myth: End-of-life care is only for the very last days of life.** As mentioned earlier, end-of-life care can be appropriate for months or even years, depending on the individual's circumstances.

- **Myth: Choosing palliative care means giving up.** Palliative care is about focusing on quality of life, not giving up. It allows individuals to live as fully and comfortably as possible in the time they have remaining.

- **Myth: Pain management at end-of-life will turn someone into a "zombie."** Modern pain management techniques can effectively control pain without necessarily impairing consciousness. The goal is to find a balance between pain relief and maintaining alertness.

- **Myth: Talking about death is taboo.** While it can be a difficult topic, open and honest communication about death and dying is essential for ensuring that an individual's wishes are respected and that their loved ones are prepared.

Understanding what end-of-life care truly means is the first step towards providing compassionate and effective support to your loved one. It's about embracing a holistic approach that addresses the physical, emotional, and spiritual needs of the individual and their family, allowing them to navigate this final stage of life with dignity, comfort, and peace. It's not about giving up hope, but rather redefining hope – hope for comfort, hope for connection, and hope for a peaceful transition.

Different Types of End-of-Life Care

The end-of-life journey is a deeply personal and often challenging experience for individuals and their families. Navigating this final chapter requires understanding the available options to make informed decisions that prioritize comfort, dignity, and quality of life.

Understanding the Spectrum of End-of-Life Care

End-of-life care encompasses a range of services and approaches designed to support individuals facing a life-limiting illness or the natural process of aging and decline.

Palliative Care: Comfort and Quality of Life at Any Stage

Palliative care is a holistic approach focusing on relieving pain and other symptoms, regardless of the stage of illness. It is appropriate for individuals of any age and at any point in a serious illness, it can be provided alongside curative treatment. Palliative care addresses physical, emotional, social, and spiritual needs, aiming to improve overall quality of life for both the patient and their family.

- **Key Components:** Symptom management, emotional and psychological support, spiritual care, social support, advance care planning, and care coordination.

- **Benefits:** Improved quality of life, reduced pain and symptoms, enhanced emotional well-being, increased patient/family satisfaction, fewer hospitalizations, and a better understanding of the illness.

Hospice Care: Comfort and Support in the Final Stages

Hospice care is a specialized type of palliative care for individuals with a terminal illness and a life expectancy of six months or less (if the illness runs its normal course). It prioritizes comfort, support, and dignity in the final stages of life, emphasizing comfort over cure.

- **Key Components:** Physician-directed care, nursing care, pain and symptom management, emotional and spiritual support, social work services, home health aide services, respite care, and bereavement support.

- **Eligibility:** Terminal illness with a life expectancy of six months or less, a desire to focus on comfort care, and a willingness to receive care at home or in a hospice facility.

- **Levels of Care:** Routine home care, continuous home care, general inpatient care, and respite care.

In-Home Care: Support in Familiar Surroundings

In-home care allows individuals to receive care in the comfort of their own homes. Services range from assistance with daily living activities to skilled nursing care. This option is particularly beneficial for those who wish to remain in a familiar environment and maintain independence.

- **Types of Services:** Personal care (bathing, dressing, grooming), homemaker services (housekeeping, meal prep), skilled nursing care (medication administration, wound care), and therapy services (physical, occupational, speech).

- **Benefits:** Remaining at home, promoting independence, personalized care, and potential cost-effectiveness compared to facility-based care.

Residential Care Facilities: Supportive Community Living

Residential care facilities (assisted living or board and care homes) provide housing, meals, and supportive services for individuals needing assistance with daily living activities but not 24-hour skilled nursing care. They offer a community environment and are suitable for those no longer able to live independently.

- **Services Offered:** Housing, meals, personal care, medication management, social activities, and transportation.

- **Benefits:** Safe and supportive environment, social interaction, and reduced burden on family caregivers.

Skilled Nursing Facilities: 24-Hour Medical Care

Skilled nursing facilities (nursing homes) provide 24-hour skilled nursing care for individuals requiring a high level of medical attention. They offer a range of services, including medical care, rehabilitation, and assistance with daily living. SNFs are often the best option for those with complex medical needs or requiring 24-hour supervision.

- **Services Offered:** 24-hour skilled nursing care, physician services, rehabilitation services, medication management, social services, and activities.

- **Benefits:** 24-hour medical care and supervision, rehabilitation services, and a supportive environment for complex medical needs.

Respite Care: A Break for Caregivers

Respite care provides temporary relief for caregivers, allowing them to take a break. It can be provided in various settings, such as at home, in an adult day care center, or in a residential facility. Prioritizing caregiver well-being and utilizing respite care is essential to prevent burnout.

- **Types of Respite Care:** In-home respite, adult day care, and overnight respite.

- **Benefits:** Reduced caregiver stress and burnout, allowing caregivers to rest and recharge, and improving the quality of care provided.

Choosing the Right Type of End-of-Life Care

The best choice depends on several factors:

- Medical condition and prognosis.
- Individual preferences and wishes.
- Required level of care.
- Available resources and support.
- Financial resources.

Open communication with the individual, their family, and the healthcare team is essential. Consider the benefits and drawbacks of each option to make a decision aligned with the individual's needs and values.

Advance Care Planning: Making Wishes Known

Advance care planning is a process involving discussions about values, goals, and preferences for future medical care. It includes creating advance directives (legal documents like living wills and durable power of attorney for healthcare) to ensure wishes are respected if the individual becomes unable to communicate.

Advance care planning is an important process that empowers individuals to make informed decisions about their future healthcare, especially when they may be unable to communicate their wishes.

It's a gift to loved ones, relieving the burden of guesswork and ensuring the person's voice is heard, even when they can't speak.

Why is Advance Care Planning Important?

Life is unpredictable. Accidents, sudden illnesses, or the natural progression of chronic conditions can leave individuals unable to express their healthcare preferences. Without advance care planning, loved ones are often left to make difficult decisions, often during highly stressful and emotional times. This can lead to:

- **Uncertainty and Stress for Families:** Family members may disagree about the best course of action, leading to conflict and added emotional burden during an already difficult time.

- **Unwanted Medical Interventions:** Without clear directives, individuals may receive medical treatments they wouldn't have wanted, potentially prolonging suffering or compromising their quality of life.

- **Loss of Autonomy:** Advance care planning preserves an individual's autonomy and right to make choices about their own body and care, even when they are no longer able to express themselves.

- **Improved End-of-Life Care:** When wishes are known, healthcare providers can provide care that aligns with the individual's values and preferences, leading to a more peaceful and dignified end-of-life experience.

Key Components of Advance Care Planning

Advance care planning involves several key steps and documents:

Reflecting on Values and Goals: This is the foundation of the process. Take time to consider what is truly important to your loved one regarding their health and well-being. What constitutes a good quality of life? What are their fears and concerns about illness and dying? What are their spiritual beliefs and how do they relate to their healthcare decisions?

Learning about Medical Options: Educate yourself about different medical treatments, procedures, and end-of-life care options. Talk to the doctor about their specific health conditions and potential future scenarios. Understanding the risks and benefits of various interventions will help them and you make informed decisions.

Choosing a Healthcare Proxy (Agent): A healthcare proxy, also known as a durable power of attorney for healthcare or healthcare agent, is a person that is designated to make medical decisions on your loved one's behalf if they become unable to do so. This person should be someone they trust implicitly, who understands their values and wishes, and who is willing to advocate for them.

Documenting Their Wishes: Advance Directives: Advance directives are legal documents that outline your loved one's healthcare preferences. The two primary types are:

- **Living Will:** A living will specifies the types of medical treatments a person wants to receive or refuse in specific situations, such as when you are terminally ill, permanently unconscious, or have an irreversible condition. It often addresses life-sustaining measures like mechanical ventilation, artificial nutrition and hydration, and cardiopulmonary resuscitation (CPR).

- **Healthcare Proxy (Durable Power of Attorney for Healthcare):** This document designates your chosen representative (proxy or agent) to make medical decisions for you when you are unable to communicate. It is broader than a living will, as it covers all medical situations, not just those outlined in the living will.

Communicating Wishes: It's not enough to simply have these documents. It's crucial to have open and honest conversations with the healthcare proxy, family members, and the doctor about your loved one's values, goals, and healthcare preferences. Make sure they understand their wishes and are comfortable with the role they will play.

Reviewing and Updating Regularly: Life circumstances, health conditions, and personal preferences can change over time. It's important to review and update the advance directives periodically, especially after a significant health event or change in their life.

Practical Steps to Get Started

- **Start the Conversation:** Initiating the conversation about end-of-life care can be challenging, but it's essential. Your loved one should start by talking to their healthcare proxy and then gradually include other family members and close friends.

- **Use Available Resources:** Numerous resources are available to guide you through the process, including:

- PREPARE for Your Care: This program offers resources and tools to help you engage in advance care planning.

- The Conversation Project: This initiative provides conversation starters and guides for discussing end-of-life care.

- National Hospice and Palliative Care Organization (NHPCO): Offers information and resources on advance care planning.

- Your State's Attorney General's Office: Often provides information and forms for advance directives.

- **Complete the Documents:** Once you have clarified your loved one's wishes, have them complete the necessary legal documents, including a living will and a healthcare proxy. Make sure these documents are easily accessible to the healthcare providers and family.

- **Talk to Your Doctor:** Discuss the advance directives with your loved one's doctor and ensure they are included in the medical record.

- **Keep the Conversation Going:** Advance care planning is an ongoing process. Continue to have conversations with your loved one and healthcare providers as circumstances change.

The Importance of Communication

Open and honest communication is vital throughout the end-of-life journey. Discussions about goals of care, treatment options, and end-of-life wishes can be difficult but are essential for making informed decisions and ensuring the individual's voice is heard.

Navigating end-of-life care can be challenging, but understanding the different options available empowers individuals and families to make informed choices that prioritize comfort, dignity, and quality of life. By engaging in open communication, utilizing available resources, and focusing on individual needs and preferences, the end-of-life journey can be approached with compassion, understanding, and peace.

Chapter 2

Understanding the Dying Process

In this chapter we will talk about the physical and emotional changes that occur during the dying process, which helps caregivers anticipate and understand what to expect.

The journey toward the end of life is a deeply personal and often mysterious experience. For caregivers, witnessing a loved one navigate this final chapter can be both profoundly moving and incredibly challenging.

Understanding the dying process, while not eliminating the emotional weight, can provide a framework for anticipating changes, offering appropriate support, and finding comfort in knowing what to expect.

The Individual Nature of Dying:

It's important to remember that every individual's experience of dying is unique. There is no single, predictable path. While some common patterns exist, the specific timing, sequence of events, and intensity of symptoms can vary significantly. Factors such as the underlying illness, age, overall health, personality, and emotional and spiritual makeup all play a role. This chapter offers general information, but it's essential to remember that your loved one's experience may differ.

Physical Changes

As the body begins to shut down, several physical changes may occur. These changes can be unsettling to witness, but understanding their nature can help alleviate fear and anxiety.

Changes in Breathing

Breathing patterns often change as death nears. It may become shallow, rapid, irregular, or labored. Periods of apnea (pauses in breathing) may occur.

Changes in breathing are a common and often unsettling part of the dying process. Several factors contribute to these shifts and understanding them can help caregivers provide better support and alleviate some of the anxiety associated with witnessing these changes.

Decreased Lung Function

As the body's systems begin to slow down, lung function can be compromised. This can be due to a variety of factors, including:

- **Weakened Respiratory Muscles:** The muscles responsible for breathing may weaken, making it harder for the lungs to expand and contract effectively.

- **Fluid Buildup:** Fluid may accumulate in the lungs, making it difficult to breathe.

- **Changes in Lung Tissue:** The structure of the lungs themselves may change due to disease or age, reducing their capacity to exchange oxygen and carbon dioxide.

Changes in the Brain's Respiratory Centers

The brain plays an important role in regulating breathing. As death approaches, changes in brain function can affect the respiratory centers, leading to irregular breathing patterns. These changes can include:

- **Reduced Blood Flow:** Decreased blood flow to the brain can affect the function of the respiratory centers.

- **Neurotransmitter Changes:** Changes in the levels of neurotransmitters, chemicals that transmit signals in the brain, can disrupt the normal regulation of breathing.

Underlying Medical Conditions

Many terminal illnesses can directly impact breathing. For example:

- **Lung Diseases:** Conditions like chronic obstructive pulmonary disease (COPD) or lung cancer can severely impair lung function.

- **Heart Failure:** A weakened heart may not be able to pump enough blood to the lungs, leading to shortness of breath.

- **Neurological Conditions:** Diseases like ALS (amyotrophic lateral sclerosis) can affect the nerves and muscles involved in breathing.

Medications

Some medications can affect breathing, particularly in individuals with compromised lung function. It's essential to discuss any medications your loved one is taking with the healthcare team to ensure they are not contributing to breathing difficulties. You need to be aware of any potential side effects, especially for those receiving end-of-life care.

Opioids:

- Opioids are powerful pain medications that can depress the central nervous system, which includes the respiratory centers in the brain.

- This can lead to slow, shallow breathing, or even respiratory arrest, especially at high doses or when combined with other central nervous system depressants.

- Examples include morphine, oxycodone, fentanyl, and codeine.

Benzodiazepines:

- Benzodiazepines are used to treat anxiety and insomnia. They also depress the central nervous system and can cause respiratory depression, particularly when taken in high doses or combined with opioids or alcohol.

- Examples include diazepam (Valium), lorazepam (Ativan), and alprazolam (Xanax).

Barbiturates:

- Barbiturates are sedatives and anticonvulsants that also depress the central nervous system. They carry a high risk of respiratory depression and are less commonly used today due to safer alternatives.

Anesthetics:

- General anesthetics used during surgery can significantly affect breathing, requiring careful monitoring and support from anesthesiologists.

Certain Antibiotics:

- Some antibiotics, such as nitrofurantoin (Macrobid), can cause lung problems and breathing difficulties, although these reactions are rare.

Heart Medications:

- Certain heart medications, like amiodarone, can cause lung damage and shortness of breath in some individuals.

Chemotherapy Drugs:

- Some chemotherapy drugs, such as bleomycin and methotrexate, can cause lung problems and breathing difficulties as a side effect.

NSAIDs:

- Nonsteroidal anti-inflammatory drugs (NSAIDs), such as aspirin and ibuprofen, can worsen asthma symptoms in some people.

Beta Blockers:

- Beta blockers, used to treat high blood pressure and other conditions, can cause wheezing in individuals with asthma or COPD.

Over-the-counter medications:

- Some over-the-counter medications, such as antihistamines (diphenhydramine) and cough suppressants (dextromethorphan), can cause drowsiness and respiratory depression, especially when taken in high doses or combined with other sedatives.

Important Considerations

- **Pre-existing Conditions:** Individuals with asthma, COPD, sleep apnea, or other respiratory conditions are at increased risk for breathing problems from these medications.

- **Dosage:** Higher doses of these medications carry a greater risk of respiratory depression.

- **Combinations:** Taking multiple medications that depress the central nervous system, such as opioids and benzodiazepines, significantly increases the risk of breathing problems.

- **Elderly:** Older adults may be more susceptible to respiratory depression from these medications due to age-related changes in metabolism and lung function.

Recommendations

- **Discuss with the doctor:** Always inform the doctor about all medications your loved one is taking, including over-the-counter drugs and supplements.

- **Follow instructions:** Take medications exactly as prescribed and do not exceed the recommended dosage.

- **Be aware of side effects:** Be aware of the potential side effects of your medications, including any breathing difficulties.

- **Report problems:** If your loved one is experiencing any breathing problems while taking medication, seek immediate medical attention.

Emotional and Psychological Factors

Anxiety and fear can also affect breathing patterns. Individuals who are anxious or afraid may breathe more rapidly or shallowly. Providing emotional support and creating a calm environment can help ease breathing difficulties.

Common Breathing Patterns

Several distinct breathing patterns may emerge as death approaches:

- **Cheyne-Stokes Respiration:** This pattern is characterized by periods of deep, rapid breathing alternating with periods of apnea (no breathing).

- **Agonal Breathing:** This involves irregular, gasping breaths that may sound labored or noisy.

- **Shallow Breathing:** Breathing may become shallow and rapid, with minimal chest movement.

Important Considerations

- **Distress:** While these breathing changes can be distressing to witness, it's important to remember that the dying person may not be aware of them or experiencing any discomfort.

- **Communication:** If your loved one is able to communicate, ask them about their breathing. They may be able to describe any sensations they are experiencing.

- **Comfort:** Work with the healthcare team to ensure your loved one is as comfortable as possible. This may involve positioning them in a way that eases breathing, using a fan to circulate air, or administering medications to manage anxiety or secretions.

Changes in Circulation

Changes in circulation are a common and often visible part of the dying process. As the body's systems begin to slow down, the circulatory system, responsible for transporting blood throughout the body, is also affected. As circulation slows down, it leads to coolness in the extremities (hands, feet, legs).

What Happens to Circulation as Death Approaches?

- **Slowing Blood Flow:** The heart, the engine of the circulatory system, may beat less forcefully and efficiently. This leads to a decrease in blood flow throughout the body.

- **Blood Redistribution:** The body prioritizes blood flow to vital organs, such as the brain and heart. This means that less blood is directed to the extremities, like the hands, feet, and legs.

- **Changes in Blood Pressure:** Blood pressure may gradually decrease as the heart's pumping ability weakens.

- **Reduced Peripheral Perfusion:** Reduced blood flow to the extremities leads to decreased peripheral perfusion, meaning the tissues in the hands and feet receive less oxygen and nutrients.

Visible Signs of Changes in Circulation

Several visible signs can indicate changes in circulation as death approaches:

- **Coolness in Extremities:** The hands, feet, and legs may feel cool or cold to the touch due to reduced blood flow.

- **Skin Color Changes:** The skin may become pale or mottled, with a bluish or purplish discoloration, especially in the extremities. This is due to decreased oxygenation of the blood and reduced blood flow to the skin's surface.

- **Weak Pulse:** The pulse may become weak, faint, or difficult to detect, particularly in the wrists and ankles.

- **Changes in Nail Beds:** The nail beds may appear pale or bluish due to reduced blood flow.

Important Considerations

- **Distress:** While these changes can be distressing to witness, it's important to remember that the dying person may not be aware of them or are experiencing any discomfort.

- **Warmth:** Even though the extremities may feel cool, avoid using excessive external heat sources, as these can cause burns or discomfort. Instead, offer blankets for warmth and comfort.

- **Positioning:** Position your loved one comfortably to promote circulation and prevent pressure sores.

- **Emotional Support:** Provide emotional support and reassurance to your loved one and their family during this time.

Working with the Healthcare Team

The healthcare team plays a crucial role in managing changes in circulation and ensuring comfort during the dying process. They can:

- **Assess Circulation:** Regularly assess circulation and monitor for any changes.

- **Manage Symptoms:** Administer medications to manage any discomfort or anxiety associated with circulatory changes.

- **Provide Education:** Offer education and support to caregivers and family members about what to expect.

Changes in Eating and Drinking

Appetite typically decreases, and the individual may lose interest in food and drink. This is a natural part of the dying process and not a sign of neglect. Forcing food or fluids can be uncomfortable and is generally not recommended.

As the body begins to shut down, its energy requirements decrease, and the ability to process food and fluids diminishes.

Why Do Changes in Eating and Drinking Occur?

- **Decreased Energy Needs:** As the body's metabolism slows down, the need for energy decreases. The body naturally requires less food and fluids to function.

- **Reduced Digestive Function:** The digestive system's ability to process food and absorb nutrients may decline. This can lead to decreased appetite, nausea, and a feeling of fullness even after consuming small amounts.

- **Weakened Muscles:** The muscles involved in chewing and swallowing may weaken, making it difficult to eat and drink. This can lead to choking or coughing.

- **Changes in Senses:** Taste and smell may become less sensitive, reducing the enjoyment of food.

- **Underlying Medical Conditions:** Certain medical conditions can affect appetite and the ability to eat and drink.

- **Medications:** Some medications can cause nausea, loss of appetite, or difficulty swallowing.

- **Dehydration:** Dehydration can contribute to decreased appetite and difficulty swallowing. However, aggressive hydration in the final stages of life may not always be beneficial and can sometimes cause discomfort.

Common Changes in Eating and Drinking

- **Decreased Appetite:** A gradual decline in appetite is common. The individual may eat less at each meal or lose interest in food altogether.

- **Reduced Fluid Intake:** Fluid intake may also decrease. The individual may only take small sips or refuse drinks altogether.

- **Difficulty Swallowing:** Swallowing may become more challenging, leading to coughing, choking, or holding food in the mouth.

- **Changes in Food Preferences:** Preferences for certain foods may change. The individual may crave different foods than usual or lose interest in previously enjoyed meals.

- **Weight Loss:** Gradual weight loss is common as the body's metabolism slows down and food intake decreases.

Important Considerations

- **It's a Natural Process:** Changes in eating and drinking are often a natural part of the dying process. It's important to remember that the body is simply requiring less sustenance.

- **Don't Force Food or Fluids:** Forcing food or fluids can cause discomfort and may even lead to aspiration (food or liquid entering the lungs).

- **Focus on Comfort:** The primary goal is to ensure comfort. Offer small amounts of favorite foods if the individual desires, but don't pressure them to eat.

- **Oral Care:** Maintain good oral hygiene to keep the mouth moist and comfortable. Use a soft toothbrush or sponge to clean the mouth and apply lip balm to prevent dryness.

- **Small Sips:** Offer small sips of fluids if the individual is able to swallow. Ice chips or frozen juice chips can be refreshing.

- **Medication Administration:** If medications are difficult to swallow, talk to the healthcare team about alternative forms, such as liquids, suppositories, or injections.

Working with the Healthcare Team

The healthcare team can provide guidance and support regarding changes in eating and drinking. They can:

- **Assess the Situation:** Evaluate the individual's ability to eat and drink and identify any underlying causes for the changes.

- **Offer Recommendations:** Provide recommendations on food and fluid choices, oral care, and medication administration.

- **Manage Symptoms:** Prescribe medications to manage nausea, pain, or other symptoms that may be affecting appetite.

- **Provide Education:** Offer education and support to caregivers and family members about what to expect and how to provide comfort.

Changes in Elimination

Bowel and bladder function may change. Constipation or incontinence can occur. Urine output may decrease. These changes are due to slowing bodily functions.

Why Do These Changes Occur?

Several factors contribute to changes in elimination as death nears:

- **Slowing Metabolism:** The body's overall metabolism slows down, affecting all systems, including the digestive and urinary tracts.

- **Decreased Food and Fluid Intake:** As appetite and thirst diminish, there's less input into the system, naturally leading to less output.

- **Weakened Muscles:** The muscles controlling bowel and bladder function may weaken, making it harder to control elimination.

- **Changes in Nervous System Function:** The nervous system, which regulates these functions, undergoes changes that can affect bowel and bladder control.

- **Underlying Medical Conditions:** Existing medical conditions can influence elimination patterns.

- **Medications:** Some medications can contribute to constipation or diarrhea.

- **Dehydration:** Dehydration can affect both bowel and bladder function.

Common Changes in Elimination

- **Constipation:** This is a frequent issue due to slowed digestion, decreased food and fluid intake, and the effects of some medications (especially pain medications).

- **Incontinence (Bowel and/or Bladder):** Loss of control over bowel or bladder function can occur due to weakened muscles and changes in nervous system function.

- **Decreased Urine Output:** As fluid intake decreases and kidney function slows, urine output naturally diminishes. Urine may also become more concentrated and darker in color.

- **Changes in Bowel Movements:** Bowel movements may become less frequent, smaller, or harder.

Important Considerations for Caregivers

- **It's a Natural Process:** Changes in elimination are often a normal part of the dying process. Try not to feel anxious or guilty about these changes.

- **Focus on Comfort and Cleanliness:** Prioritize keeping your loved one clean, comfortable, and dry. This helps prevent skin breakdown and promotes dignity.

- **Regular Checks:** Check frequently for bowel movements or the need to urinate, especially if your loved one is unable to communicate their needs.

- **Skin Care:** Pay close attention to skin care, especially in incontinent individuals, to prevent pressure sores and skin irritation. Cleanse the skin gently after each episode of incontinence and apply a barrier cream if necessary.

- **Hydration:** While it's important to ensure adequate hydration, especially if constipation is a problem, consult with the healthcare team about appropriate fluid intake. Overhydration can sometimes cause discomfort in the final stages of life.

- **Medication Management:** Discuss any concerns about constipation or diarrhea with the healthcare team. They can recommend appropriate medications or strategies.

- **Dignity and Respect:** Approach these intimate caregiving tasks with sensitivity, respect, and understanding. Maintain your loved one's dignity by providing privacy and minimizing any embarrassment they might feel.

Working with the Healthcare Team

The healthcare team is a valuable resource for managing elimination issues during the dying process. They can:

- **Assess the Situation:** Evaluate your loved one's bowel and bladder function and identify any contributing factors to changes in elimination.

- **Provide Recommendations:** Offer guidance on managing constipation, incontinence, and other elimination problems.

- **Prescribe Medications:** Prescribe stool softeners, laxatives, or other medications as needed.

- **Provide Education and Support:** Educate caregivers and family members about what to expect and how to provide appropriate care.

Changes in Consciousness

The level of consciousness may fluctuate. The individual may become drowsy, confused, disoriented, or unresponsive. Periods of lucidity may occur even as death approaches. These changes are often due to changes in brain function.

Why Do Changes in Consciousness Occur?

Several factors contribute to changes in consciousness as death nears:

- **Changes in Brain Function:** As the body's systems begin to shut down, the brain's function is affected. This can be due to reduced blood flow, changes in brain chemistry, or the effects of the underlying illness.

- **Medications:** Some medications, particularly those used for pain management, can affect consciousness.

- **Dehydration:** Dehydration can contribute to confusion and decreased alertness.

- **Organ Failure:** If vital organs, such as the liver or kidneys, begin to fail, toxins can build up in the body and affect brain function.

- **Underlying Medical Conditions:** Certain medical conditions, such as dementia or brain tumors, can directly impact consciousness.

Common Changes in Consciousness

- **Drowsiness:** The individual may become increasingly drowsy, spending more time asleep and being difficult to arouse.

- **Confusion:** Confusion, disorientation, and difficulty recognizing people or places can occur.

- **Restlessness or Agitation:** Some individuals may become restless, agitated, or even combative. This can be due to pain, discomfort, or changes in brain function.

- **Delirium:** Delirium, a state of confusion and disorientation, can occur. It may involve hallucinations or vivid dreams.

- **Periods of Lucidity:** Even as death approaches, there may be periods of lucidity when the individual is more alert and able to communicate. These moments can be precious opportunities for connection.

- **Unresponsiveness:** Eventually, the individual may become completely unresponsive, unable to communicate or react to their surroundings.

Important Considerations for Caregivers

- **It's a Natural Part of the Process:** Changes in consciousness are often a natural part of the dying process. It's important to remember that these changes are not a reflection of the care being provided.

- **Communication:** Even if your loved one seems unresponsive, continue to talk to them. Hearing is often the last sense to go, so they may still be able to hear your voice and feel your presence.

- **Presence:** Simply being present with your loved one, holding their hand, and offering words of love and support can be profoundly comforting, even if they are not fully conscious.

- **Comfort:** Ensure your loved one is as comfortable as possible. This may involve managing pain, adjusting their position, or providing a calm and peaceful environment.

- **Reassurance:** If your loved one is agitated or restless, try to reassure them and create a calming atmosphere. Talk to the healthcare team about medications that may help manage these symptoms.

- **Respect:** Respect your loved one's wishes regarding end-of-life care, including any advance directives they may have.

Working with the Healthcare Team

The healthcare team can provide valuable support and guidance regarding changes in consciousness. They can:

- **Assess the Situation:** Evaluate the individual's level of consciousness and identify any contributing factors to the changes.

- **Manage Symptoms:** Prescribe medications to manage pain, agitation, or delirium.

- **Provide Education:** Educate caregivers and family members about what to expect and how to provide appropriate care.

- **Offer Emotional Support:** Offer emotional support to caregivers and family members as they navigate this challenging time.

Terminal Lucidity

Terminal lucidity is a fascinating and somewhat mysterious phenomenon where a person with a severe mental illness or cognitive impairment experiences a sudden, temporary period of mental clarity and awareness shortly before death. It's like a brief window in time where they seem to "wake up" and regain cognitive abilities they may have lost years ago.

Here's what we know about terminal lucidity:

- **It's unexpected:** It often occurs in individuals with conditions like Alzheimer's disease, dementia, or schizophrenia, where cognitive decline is progressive and seemingly irreversible. The sudden return of clarity is unexpected and often occurs close to the time of death.

- **It's temporary:** The period of lucidity is brief, lasting anywhere from a few minutes to a few hours. It's not a sustained improvement, and the person typically returns to their previous cognitive state before death.

- **It's not fully understood:** The causes of terminal lucidity are not fully understood. Several theories exist, including changes in brain chemistry, a surge of brain activity, or even a spiritual or psychological component. More research is needed to understand the underlying mechanisms.

- **It's not a sign of recovery:** While witnessing a loved one experience terminal lucidity can be a beautiful and bittersweet moment, it's important to remember that it's not a sign of recovery. It's often a sign that death is near.

What might you observe during terminal lucidity?

- **Improved communication:** A person who has been unable to speak coherently may suddenly be able to communicate clearly, express their needs, or share their thoughts and feelings.

- **Recognition of loved ones:** They may recognize and interact with family members or friends they haven't recognized in a long time.

- **Recollection of memories:** They might recall and share memories from the past, even long-forgotten ones.

- **Emotional expression:** They may express a range of emotions, such as love, gratitude, or regret.

What should you do if you witness terminal lucidity?

- **Be present:** The most important thing is to be present with your loved one and cherish these precious moments of clarity.

- **Listen attentively:** Give them your full attention and listen to what they have to say.

- **Offer comfort and support:** Provide emotional support and reassurance. Let them know you are there for them.

- **Respect their wishes:** If they express any wishes or needs, do your best to honor them.

- **Acknowledge the moment:** Recognize the significance of this moment and allow yourself to experience the emotions that come with it.

Terminal lucidity can be a profound and meaningful experience for both the dying person and their loved ones.

It can provide an opportunity for connection, closure, and the expression of love and gratitude. While the phenomenon remains somewhat mysterious, it serves as a reminder of the complex and multifaceted nature of the human experience, even in the face of death.

Changes in Senses

While hearing is often the last sense to go, other senses may become diminished. Vision may blur, and the individual may lose interest in watching television or reading. Touch may become less sensitive.

As death approaches, a person's senses may undergo significant changes. These shifts can be subtle or more pronounced.

Common Changes in Senses:

- **Hearing:** Hearing is often the last sense to remain functional. Even when a person seems unresponsive, they may still be able to hear what is being said. This is why it's important to continue speaking to your loved one, even if they don't appear to be listening.

- **Vision:** Vision may become blurred or diminished. The person may lose interest in watching television or reading. Their eyes may appear glassy or teary, and they may have difficulty focusing.

- **Touch:** Sensitivity to touch may decrease. The person may not feel a gentle touch as readily as before. However, they may still find comfort in light touch or holding hands.

- **Taste and Smell:** The senses of taste and smell may become less sensitive. This can contribute to a decreased appetite as food may not seem as appealing as it once did.

Important Considerations for Caregivers

- **Awareness:** Even if your loved one seems withdrawn or unresponsive, it's important to assume they can still perceive their surroundings through some of their senses.

- **Communication:** Continue to talk to your loved one in a normal voice, even if they don't seem to be responding. Share memories, express your love, and offer reassurance.

- **Gentle Touch:** Offer gentle touch, such as holding their hand or stroking their arm. This can provide comfort and a sense of connection.

- **Sensory Stimulation:** Consider gentle sensory stimulation, such as playing soft music, displaying familiar photos, or using a diffuser with calming scents (if appropriate and tolerated).

- **Environment:** Create a calm and peaceful environment by dimming lights, minimizing noise, and ensuring the room is a comfortable temperature.

- **Respect:** Respect your loved one's preferences regarding sensory stimulation. If they seem overwhelmed or agitated, reduce the level of stimulation.

Working with the Healthcare Team

The healthcare team can provide guidance and support regarding changes in senses. They can:

- **Assess Sensory Function:** Evaluate the individual's sensory abilities and identify any specific challenges they are experiencing.

- **Offer Recommendations:** Provide recommendations on how to adapt the environment and provide sensory stimulation in a way that is comfortable and appropriate.

- **Manage Symptoms:** If the individual is experiencing any discomfort or distress related to sensory changes, the healthcare team can offer interventions to manage these symptoms.

Changes in Muscle Tone

Changes in muscle tone are a common and often visible part of the dying process. As the body begins to shut down, the muscles, like other systems, are affected. Muscles may become weak and relaxed. This can lead to difficulty with movement, swallowing, and maintaining posture.

What Happens to Muscle Tone?

- **Muscle Weakness:** The muscles throughout the body gradually weaken. This can lead to difficulty with movement, such as turning in bed, sitting up, or even holding the head up.

- **Loss of Muscle Tone:** Muscles may become flaccid or lose their tone. This can result in a slack or drooping appearance.

- **Decreased Reflexes:** Reflexes, which are involuntary muscle responses, may become diminished or absent.

- **Difficulty with Swallowing:** The muscles involved in swallowing may weaken, making it harder to eat and drink. This can lead to coughing, choking, or holding food in the mouth.

- **Changes in Facial Expression:** Facial muscles may weaken, leading to a drooping or slack appearance in the face.

Important Considerations

- **It's a Natural Process:** Muscle weakness and loss of muscle tone are often a natural part of the dying process. It's important to remember that these changes are not a reflection of the care being provided.

- **Comfort:** Focus on ensuring your loved one is as comfortable as possible. This may involve adjusting their position in bed, using pillows for support, or providing gentle massage.

- **Safety:** Due to muscle weakness, individuals may be at increased risk for falls or injuries. Take precautions to ensure their safety, such as assisting with movement and keeping the environment clutter-free.

- **Swallowing Difficulties:** If your loved one is having difficulty swallowing, offer small bites of soft foods or liquids. Talk to the healthcare team about alternative ways to ensure they are getting adequate nutrition and hydration.

- **Communication:** Even if your loved one is unable to speak, continue to communicate with them. They may still be able to hear your voice and feel your presence.

Working with the Healthcare Team

The healthcare team can provide valuable support and guidance regarding changes in muscle tone. They can:

- **Assess Muscle Function:** Evaluate the individual's muscle strength and identify any specific challenges they are experiencing.

- **Offer Recommendations:** Provide recommendations on how to support movement, prevent falls, and manage any difficulties with swallowing.

- **Manage Symptoms:** If the individual is experiencing any discomfort or pain related to muscle weakness, the healthcare team can offer interventions to manage these symptoms.

Emotional and Spiritual Changes

The dying process is not only physical but also deeply emotional and spiritual. Individuals may experience a range of emotions, including:

- **Fear and Anxiety:** Fear of the unknown, fear of pain, and anxiety about leaving loved ones are common.

- **Sadness and Grief:** Grief for lost abilities, lost relationships, and the impending loss of life.

- **Anger and Frustration:** Anger at the illness, frustration with the limitations it imposes, and resentment at the unfairness of the situation.

- **Acceptance and Peace:** As death approaches, some individuals may experience a sense of acceptance and peace, finding comfort in their faith or in the love and support of their family.

- **Spiritual Reflection:** This can be a time of deep spiritual reflection, as individuals contemplate the meaning of life, their relationships, and their legacy.

Supporting Your Loved One

Understanding the dying process allows caregivers to provide more effective and compassionate support.

- **Physical Comfort:** Focus on managing symptoms and ensuring physical comfort. This may involve working with the healthcare team to administer pain medication, provide personal care, and create a comfortable environment.

- **Emotional Support:** Offer emotional support by listening attentively, validating feelings, and providing reassurance. Create a safe space for your loved one to express their fears, anxieties, and hopes.

- **Spiritual Support:** Respect and honor your loved one's spiritual beliefs and practices. This may involve connecting them with a chaplain or spiritual advisor, reading sacred texts, or simply providing a quiet space for reflection.

- **Presence and Connection:** The most important thing you can offer your loved one is your presence. Simply being there, holding their hand, and offering words of love and support can be profoundly comforting.

The Importance of the Healthcare Team

The healthcare team plays a vital role in supporting both the individual and their family during the dying process. They can:

- **Provide Education:** Offer information about the dying process and what to expect.

- **Manage Symptoms:** Provide expert symptom management to maximize comfort.

- **Offer Emotional and Spiritual Support:** Provide counseling, support groups, and spiritual care services.

- **Coordinate Care:** Coordinate care among different healthcare providers to ensure seamless and comprehensive support.

Remembering the Individual

While the physical and emotional changes of the dying process can be challenging to witness, it's important to remember the individual behind the illness. Focus on celebrating their life, sharing memories, and expressing love and gratitude. These moments of connection can be deeply meaningful for both the dying person and their loved ones.

Understanding the dying process is not about predicting the exact course of events, but rather about preparing yourself emotionally and practically for the changes that may occur. It's about recognizing the individual's unique journey and providing compassionate support that honors their dignity, respects their wishes, and celebrates their life. By embracing this understanding, caregivers can navigate this challenging time with greater confidence, compassion, and peace.

Chapter 3

Recognizing Signs and Symptoms

Identifying key indicators of approaching death, including physical changes, altered consciousness, and emotional withdrawal. This chapter will help caregivers prepare and manage expectations.

The Variability of the Dying Process

Every individual's experience is unique. It's a fundamental truth that every individual's experience of dying is unique, shaped by a multitude of factors. This variability makes it challenging to predict exactly how someone will transition in their final stages of life, but it also underscores the importance of personalized care and support.

Here's a breakdown of why the dying process is so variable:

Underlying Health Conditions

- **Type of Illness:** Different diseases progress in different ways. Cancer, heart failure, dementia, and other illnesses have distinct trajectories with varying timelines and symptom patterns.

- **Severity of Illness:** The stage and severity of the underlying illness significantly influence the dying process. Someone with advanced cancer may experience a different trajectory than someone with early-stage heart failure.

- **Co-existing Conditions:** Individuals often have multiple health conditions, which can interact and complicate the dying process.

Individual Factors

- **Age:** Age plays a role, as younger individuals may experience the dying process differently than older adults.

- **Overall Health:** A person's general health and fitness level before the terminal illness can influence how their body responds as death approaches.

- **Physical and Emotional Resilience:** Some individuals may possess greater physical or emotional resilience, which can affect their ability to cope with the challenges of dying.

- **Personality and Coping Style:** A person's personality and how they typically cope with stress and adversity can shape their emotional and psychological experience of dying.

Emotional and Spiritual Factors

- **Emotional State:** Unresolved emotional issues, fears, or anxieties can influence the dying process.

- **Spiritual Beliefs:** Spiritual beliefs and practices can provide comfort and meaning during the dying process.

- **Relationships and Support System:** Strong relationships and a supportive network of family and friends can significantly impact a person's emotional and psychological well-being as death approaches.

Care and Treatment

- **Access to Care:** The quality and availability of healthcare services, including palliative care and hospice, can influence a person's comfort and overall experience.

- **Pain Management:** Effective pain and symptom management can significantly impact a person's comfort and quality of life during the dying process.

- **Medications:** Medications can have both intended and unintended effects on the dying process, influencing consciousness, comfort, and other symptoms.

The Unknown

- **The Mystery of Death:** Despite advances in medicine, there is still much we don't understand about the process of dying. It remains a deeply personal and often mysterious experience.

Implications for Caregivers

- **Embrace Uncertainty:** It's important to accept that there will be uncertainties and variations in your loved one's dying process.

- **Focus on the Present:** Rather than trying to predict the future, focus on providing comfort and support in the present moment.

- **Individualized Care:** Tailor your caregiving approach to your loved one's specific needs, preferences, and wishes.

- **Open Communication:** Maintain open and honest communication with your loved one, their healthcare team, and other family members.

- **Seek Support:** Don't hesitate to seek support from healthcare professionals, counselors, or support groups for yourself and your family.

The difference between "actively dying" and a longer terminal phase

It's important to understand the difference between the terminal phase and the actively dying phase, as it can help caregivers and families prepare for what to expect.

Terminal Phase

- This is the period when a person is living with a terminal illness and is no longer responding to curative treatment.

- It can last for weeks, months, or even years.

- During this time, the person may experience a gradual decline in physical and cognitive function.

- They may still be able to engage in activities and interact with loved ones, although their abilities may be limited.

Actively Dying Phase

- This is the final stage of the dying process, when the body is actively shutting down.

- It typically lasts for a few days or hours.

- During this time, the person will experience significant changes in physical and cognitive function.

- They may become unresponsive, have difficulty breathing, and experience changes in circulation.

Key Differences

Feature	Terminal Phase	Actively Dying Phase
Duration	Weeks, months, or years	Days or hours
Physical Function	Gradual decline	Significant decline
Cognitive Function	May be impaired, but some interaction is possible	Often unresponsive
Breathing	May be labored or irregular	Often shallow, gasping, or periods of apnea
Circulation	Cool extremities, but skin color may be normal	Mottled or bluish skin, especially extremities
Eating and Drinking	Decreased appetite and fluid intake	Refusal of food and fluids
Elimination	Changes in bowel and bladder function	Incontinence

Recognizing the Signs

It's important to remember that everyone experiences the dying process differently. However, some common signs that a person is actively dying include:

- Changes in breathing, such as Cheyne-Stokes respiration or agonal breathing
- Cool, clammy skin
- Mottling or bluish discoloration of the skin
- Decreased urine output
- Incontinence
- Loss of consciousness
- Noisy breathing or "death rattle"

What to Do

If you believe your loved one is actively dying, it's important to:

- Contact their healthcare team or hospice provider.
- Focus on providing comfort and support.
- Continue to talk to them and offer reassurance.
- Respect their wishes regarding end-of-life care.

Remember

- The actively dying phase is a natural part of the dying process.

- It's important to focus on providing comfort and support during this time.

- Don't hesitate to reach out to healthcare professionals for guidance and support.

The importance of focusing on comfort and quality of life.

As the body's systems begin to shut down, aggressive medical interventions often become more burdensome than beneficial. Continuing treatments that aim to cure may cause unnecessary suffering without significantly extending life. At this stage, the priority becomes minimizing pain and other distressing symptoms, allowing the individual to experience their final days or hours with as much peace and dignity as possible.

What Does Focusing on Comfort and Quality of Life Involve?

- **Pain Management:** This is often the most critical aspect of comfort care. Effective pain relief allows the individual to be more present and engaged, even if only for short periods. The goal is not necessarily to eliminate all pain, but to manage it to a tolerable level that allows for some degree of comfort and interaction.

- **Symptom Management:** Beyond pain, other symptoms like nausea, shortness of breath, restlessness, and anxiety can significantly impact quality of life. Addressing these symptoms with appropriate medications and non-medical interventions (e.g., positioning, relaxation techniques) is essential.

- **Emotional and Spiritual Support:** The dying process is not only physical but also deeply emotional and spiritual. Providing a safe space for the individual to express their fears, anxieties, regrets, or hopes is crucial. Offering spiritual support, whether through religious practices, connection with a chaplain, or simply providing a quiet and reflective environment, can bring comfort and peace.

- **Personal Care:** Maintaining hygiene and cleanliness is important for both physical comfort and a sense of dignity. Gentle bathing, oral care, and dressing the individual in comfortable clothing can contribute to their well-being.

- **Creating a Peaceful Environment:** Minimizing noise, dimming lights, and creating a calm and soothing atmosphere can promote relaxation and reduce anxiety. Playing soft music or displaying cherished photos can also provide comfort.

- **Meaningful Connections:** Encourage visits from loved ones and facilitate opportunities for meaningful connections. Sharing memories, expressing love and gratitude, and simply being present can be profoundly comforting for both the dying person and their family.

- **Respecting Wishes:** It's essential to honor the individual's wishes regarding end-of-life care. This includes respecting their advance directives, such as a living will or durable power of attorney for healthcare, and making decisions that align with their values and preferences.

How Caregivers Can Implement Comfort Care:

- **Work Closely with the Healthcare Team:** Open communication with doctors, nurses, and hospice professionals is vital. They can provide guidance on pain and symptom management, offer emotional support, and help navigate the practical aspects of end-of-life care.

- **Advocate for Your Loved One:** Be your loved one's voice, ensuring their needs are being met and their wishes are respected.

- **Be Present:** The most valuable gift you can give is your presence. Simply being there and offering words of love and support can be profoundly comforting.

- **Focus on the Moment:** Try to let go of anxieties about the future and focus on the present moment. Cherish the time you have together and make the most of each precious moment.

- **Take Care of Yourself:** Caregiving during this time can be emotionally and physically demanding. Remember to prioritize your own well-being by getting enough rest, eating healthy meals, and seeking support from others.

As a person is actively dying, the focus shifts from quantity of life to quality of life. By prioritizing comfort, managing symptoms, providing emotional and spiritual support, and honoring their wishes, caregivers can help their loved ones experience a peaceful and dignified end-of-life journey. It's a time for love, connection, and letting go.

Recognizing the Imminence of Death

- Intensification of physical symptoms.

- The "surge" before the calm (a brief period of increased energy or alertness, which doesn't always happen).

- The final moments: shallow breaths, slow heartbeat, loss of reflexes, cessation of breathing and heartbeat.

This list covers a broad range of potential signs and symptoms. It's crucial to remember that not everyone will experience all of these, and the order and intensity of these changes can vary greatly. Consulting with healthcare professionals is essential for accurate assessment and personalized care.

Chapter 4

The Importance of Communication

I can't Emphasize enough, the value of open and honest communication with your dying loved one, family members, and the healthcare team. This includes covering sensitive topics like discussing wishes and fears.

It's the bridge that connects everyone involved, ensuring that the dying person's wishes are honored, their needs are met, and everyone feels supported during this challenging time.

Why communication with your loved one, the healthcare team, and family is so important

Communicating with a loved one at the end of life can be a deeply meaningful experience, even when their ability to communicate changes. It's about finding ways to connect, express love, and honor their presence in whatever form that takes.

Verbal Communication

- **Speak Clearly and Slowly:** Even if your loved one is weak, speak in a normal tone of voice, clearly and slowly. Avoid shouting or speaking too quickly.

- **Simple Language:** Use simple, straightforward language and avoid complex sentences or jargon.

- **Direct Questions:** Ask direct, closed-ended questions (yes/no or one-word answers) if your loved one has difficulty formulating sentences.

- **Listen Patiently:** Give your loved one ample time to respond. Be patient and allow for pauses. Don't interrupt or try to finish their sentences.

- **Repeat and Rephrase:** If necessary, repeat or rephrase your questions or statements to ensure clarity.

- **Share Memories:** Reminisce about shared experiences, happy memories, and meaningful moments. This can bring comfort and connection.

- **Express Love and Gratitude:** Tell your loved one how much you love them and how grateful you are for their presence in your life. Don't hesitate to express your feelings openly and often.

Nonverbal Communication

Understanding the Cause of Nonverbal Communication

- **Acquired:** If nonverbal communication is due to an injury, illness (like a stroke or dementia), or progressive condition, their previous communication abilities might offer clues or a starting point.

- **Temporary:** Some conditions or treatments might temporarily affect speech. Understanding the cause can help you anticipate changes and adapt.

Observing and Interpreting Body Language

- **Facial Expressions:** Pay close attention to facial expressions. Smiles, frowns, raised eyebrows, and other expressions can convey a wide range of emotions.

- **Body Posture:** Observe body posture. Open posture often indicates receptiveness, while crossed arms or a turned body might suggest discomfort or disinterest.

- **Gestures:** Notice any gestures the person uses, even if they seem small or unintentional. These could be attempts to communicate.

- **Eye Contact:** If the person makes eye contact, it can signal engagement and a desire to connect.

- **Vocalizations:** Even if words aren't used, pay attention to any sounds the person makes, like sighs, grunts, or changes in tone. These can convey emotions or needs.

Utilizing Assistive Communication Tools

- **Communication Boards/Books:** These contain pictures, symbols, or words that the person can point to in order to express themselves.

- **Assistive Technology:** Explore apps and devices that can translate text to speech or allow communication through eye-tracking or other input methods.

- **Sign Language:** If the person knows sign language, learn some basic signs to facilitate communication. Even a few signs can make a difference.

- **Written Communication:** If the person can write, provide a notebook and pen or a digital device for them to express themselves.

Adapting Your Communication Style

- **Speak Directly:** Even if the person doesn't respond verbally, speak to them directly, not about them in the third person.

- **Use Simple Language:** Use short, clear sentences and avoid complex vocabulary or jargon.

- **Ask Closed-Ended Questions:** Questions that can be answered with a "yes" or "no" or a simple gesture can be easier to understand.

- **Offer Choices:** Instead of asking open-ended questions, offer choices. For example, "Would you like a drink of water or juice?"

- **Be Patient:** Allow plenty of time for the person to respond. Don't rush or interrupt them.

- **Repeat and Rephrase:** If you're unsure if you've understood, repeat what you think they've communicated and ask if you're correct. Rephrase your questions if necessary.

Creating a Supportive Environment

- **Minimize Distractions:** Reduce noise and other distractions to help the person focus.

- **Be Present:** Give the person your full attention and be present in the moment.

- **Respect Their Pace:** Allow them to communicate at their own pace. Don't pressure them to respond if they seem tired or overwhelmed.

- **Offer Encouragement:** Offer positive reinforcement and encouragement to build their confidence and motivation to communicate.

Working with Professionals

- **Speech-Language Pathologists (SLPs):** SLPs are trained to assess communication abilities and recommend appropriate strategies and tools.

- **Occupational Therapists (OTs):** OTs can help with adapting the environment and finding assistive devices to support communication.

- **Caregivers and Support Staff:** Communicate regularly with other caregivers and support staff to share information and ensure consistency in communication approaches.

Understanding Individual Preferences

- **Learn Their Communication Style:** Each nonverbal person has their own unique way of communicating. Take the time to learn their individual cues and preferences.

- **Observe and Document:** Keep track of what communication methods seem most effective and any patterns you notice in their responses.

Adapting to Changing Abilities

- **If Speech is Difficult**

  o **Writing:** Offer a notebook and pen or a communication board if your loved one is still able to write.

  o **Gestures:** Encourage the use of gestures or sign language if they are familiar with them.

  o **Picture Boards:** Create a picture board with common items, needs, or phrases that your loved one can point to.

- **If Cognition is Impaired**

  o **Focus on Emotions:** Even if your loved one doesn't understand your words, they may still be able to sense your emotions. Speak with warmth and love, and convey your presence through touch and facial expressions.

  o **Sensory Stimulation:** Engage their senses with gentle music, soft lighting, familiar scents (if appropriate), or by displaying cherished photos.

  o **Music Therapy:** Music can be a powerful way to connect and evoke memories, even when verbal communication is limited.

Honoring Their Preferences

- **Respect Their Pace:** Allow your loved one to communicate at their own pace. Don't rush or pressure them.

- **Honor Their Wishes:** Respect their preferences regarding communication. If they don't feel like talking or interacting, simply be present and offer your support.

- **Be Patient:** Communication can take time, especially when someone is ill or nearing the end of life. Be patient and allow the process to unfold naturally.

Maintaining open communication with your loved one during end-of-life care is essential, even when their ability to communicate changes. It's about preserving connection, honoring their dignity, and ensuring their voice is heard, however that may manifest.

Creating a Safe and Supportive Environment

- **Physical Comfort:** Ensure your loved one is as comfortable as possible. Manage pain and other symptoms, adjust their position, and create a calm and peaceful atmosphere. Physical comfort can facilitate emotional openness.

- **Emotional Safety:** Offer a safe space for them to express their feelings without judgment. Encourage them to share their fears, anxieties, hopes, and regrets. Let them know it's okay to talk about death and dying.

- **Active Listening:** Practice active listening. Give them your full attention, make eye contact (if they are able to), and avoid interrupting. Show that you are truly present and engaged in the conversation.

- **Honoring Their Wishes:** Open and honest conversations allow your loved one to express their preferences regarding end-of-life care, including medical decisions, pain management, and where they want to spend their final days. This ensures their autonomy and dignity are respected.

- **Providing Emotional Support:** Active listening and open communication create a safe space for your loved one to share their fears, anxieties, hopes, and regrets. This can bring comfort, reduce emotional distress, and facilitate a sense of closure.

- **Maintaining Connection:** Even when communication becomes difficult due to illness or cognitive decline, finding ways to connect – through touch, shared memories, or simply being present – is vital. Continue to talk to them, share your love, and offer reassurance.

- **Understanding Their Needs:** Your loved one may still be able to communicate their needs, even nonverbally. Pay attention to their body language, facial expressions, and subtle cues to understand their comfort level and any unmet needs.

Adapting to Changing Communication Abilities

- **Verbal Communication:** Even if speech becomes difficult, encourage them to speak when they feel able. Be patient and allow them time to express themselves. Ask clarifying questions gently and avoid putting words in their mouth.

- **Nonverbal Communication:** Pay close attention to nonverbal cues, such as facial expressions, body language, and gestures. These can communicate a lot, even when words are absent.

- **Written Communication:** If speaking is too difficult, offer alternative ways to communicate, such as writing notes, using a communication board, or pointing to pictures or words.

- **Touch:** Physical touch, like holding hands, stroking their arm, or giving a gentle massage, can be a powerful form of communication and connection. It can convey love, comfort, and support.

- **Shared Activities:** Engaging in shared activities, like listening to music, looking at photos, or simply being present together, can foster connection and create opportunities for nonverbal communication.

Addressing Emotional and Spiritual Needs

- **Spiritual Support:** If your loved one has spiritual beliefs, support them in connecting with their faith or spiritual community. This can provide comfort and meaning during this time.

- **Emotional Support:** Offer emotional support by acknowledging their feelings and validating their experiences. Let them know you are there for them and that they are not alone.

- **Reminiscence:** Sharing memories and stories can be a meaningful way to connect and reminisce about shared experiences. This can bring joy and comfort during the end-of-life journey.

- **Expressing Love and Gratitude:** Don't hesitate to express your love and gratitude. Tell them how much they mean to you and how much you appreciate them. These expressions can be deeply comforting for both of you.

Communication with the Healthcare Team

- **Coordinated Care:** Effective communication with doctors, nurses, and other healthcare professionals ensures coordinated and comprehensive care. Sharing information about your loved one's condition, symptoms, and preferences allows the healthcare team to provide the best possible care.

- **Informed Decision-Making:** Open communication with the healthcare team allows you to make informed decisions about medical treatments, pain management, and other aspects of care. Ask questions, clarify any doubts, and actively participate in the decision-making process.

- **Symptom Management:** Clearly communicating your loved one's symptoms – pain levels, nausea, breathing difficulties, etc. – allows the healthcare team to adjust medications and other interventions to maximize comfort.

- **Advocacy:** You are your loved one's advocate. Effective communication with the healthcare team ensures their voice is heard and their wishes are respected.

Building a Strong Foundation from the Start

- **Establish a Relationship:** From the initial diagnosis or recognition of a terminal illness, aim to build a positive and respectful relationship with the healthcare team. This includes doctors, nurses, social workers, and other involved professionals.

- **Identify a Point Person:** If possible, designate one family member or caregiver as the primary point of contact for communication with the healthcare team. This helps streamline information and avoids confusion.

- **Share Relevant Information:** Provide the healthcare team with a comprehensive medical history, including current medications, allergies, past treatments, and any relevant information about your loved one's overall health and well-being.

Proactive Communication Strategies

- **Regular Updates:** Keep the healthcare team informed about any changes in your loved one's condition, including new symptoms, changes in existing symptoms, or any concerns you may have. Don't hesitate to reach out, even if you're unsure if something is significant.

- **Prepare for Appointments:** Before each appointment, prepare a list of questions, concerns, and topics you want to discuss. This helps you stay focused and make the most of your time with the healthcare team.

- **Take Detailed Notes:** During appointments, take thorough notes about diagnoses, treatment plans, medication instructions, and any other important information shared. This will help you remember details and share information with other family members or caregivers.

- **Ask Clarifying Questions:** Don't hesitate to ask questions if you don't understand something. Medical terminology can be confusing, so it's crucial to seek clarification until you're comfortable with the information.

- **Be Specific:** When describing symptoms or concerns, be as specific as possible. Instead of saying "They're not doing well," describe specific changes you've observed, such as "They've been more lethargic in the past few days and their appetite has decreased significantly."

- **Active Listening:** Listen attentively to the healthcare team's explanations and recommendations. Show respect for their expertise and ask clarifying questions when needed.

Utilizing Available Communication Channels

- **Phone Calls:** Use phone calls for urgent matters or quick updates. Be prepared to leave a message if necessary and ensure the healthcare team has your contact information.

- **Email:** Email can be useful for non-urgent communication or sharing detailed information. However, be mindful of privacy and avoid sharing sensitive medical information via unsecured email.

- **Patient Portals:** Many healthcare systems offer online patient portals where you can communicate with the healthcare team, access medical records, and schedule appointments.

- **In-Person Meetings:** Schedule regular meetings with the healthcare team to discuss your loved one's care plan, address any concerns, and make collaborative decisions.

Addressing Challenges and Difficult Conversations

- **Differing Opinions:** If you have concerns or disagree with a recommended treatment plan, respectfully express your concerns and seek further information or a second opinion. Open communication is key to resolving disagreements.

- **Emotional Conversations:** End-of-life care often involves difficult conversations about prognosis, treatment options, and end-of-life wishes. Be prepared to discuss these sensitive topics openly and honestly with the healthcare team.

- **Cultural Sensitivity:** Be mindful of cultural differences that may influence communication styles or attitudes toward death and dying.

Maintaining a Collaborative Approach

- **Partnership:** View the healthcare team as partners in your loved one's care. Work collaboratively to develop a care plan that meets their individual needs and preferences.

- **Mutual Respect:** Treat the healthcare team with respect and courtesy. Recognize their expertise and the demands of their profession.

- **Express Gratitude:** Acknowledge and appreciate the healthcare team's efforts and support. A simple thank you can go a long way.

Communication with Family

- **Shared Understanding:** Open communication among family members ensures everyone is on the same page regarding the loved one's condition, care plan, and end-of-life wishes. This reduces misunderstandings and potential conflicts.

- **Emotional Support:** Sharing feelings, concerns, and grief with family members provides emotional support and helps everyone cope with the situation. It can also strengthen family bonds during this difficult time.

- **Collaborative Caregiving:** Effective communication among family members facilitates collaborative caregiving. Sharing responsibilities, coordinating schedules, and supporting each other can ease the burden of caregiving.

- **Decision-Making:** Family discussions can be invaluable in making difficult decisions about end-of-life care, especially when the dying person is no longer able to express their wishes.

Creating a Foundation of Openness

- **Early and Honest Conversations:** Ideally, discussions about end-of-life care should begin well before a crisis. This allows family members time to process information, share their feelings, and participate in planning.

- **Regular Updates:** Keep family members informed about your loved one's condition, any changes in their care plan, and upcoming decisions. Regular updates, even if there's no "news," can help everyone feel connected and involved.

- **Designated Communication Person:** If possible, designate one family member (or a close friend) as the primary point of contact for sharing information. This helps streamline communication and prevents confusion.

Facilitating Meaningful Discussions

- **Family Meetings:** Organize family meetings to discuss important topics related to end-of-life care. These meetings provide a structured forum for sharing information, expressing concerns, and making decisions together.

- **Shared Decision-Making:** Encourage all family members to participate in decision-making, as appropriate. Value everyone's input and strive for consensus, even when there are differing opinions.

- **Active Listening:** Practice active listening during family discussions. Give each person a chance to speak without interruption and show genuine interest in their perspectives.

- **Respectful Dialogue:** Encourage respectful dialogue, even when there are disagreements. Remind everyone that the shared goal is to provide the best possible care for your loved one.

Utilizing Effective Communication Strategies

- **Multiple Communication Channels:** Use a variety of communication channels to keep family members informed. This might include phone calls, emails, text messages, video conferencing, or a shared online platform.

- **Written Summaries:** After family meetings or important discussions, send out a written summary of key points and decisions made. This helps ensure everyone is on the same page and provides a record of the conversation.

- **Visual Aids:** Visual aids such as charts or diagrams can be helpful for explaining complex medical information or care plans.

- **One-on-One Conversations:** In addition to group discussions, make time for one-on-one conversations with individual family members. This allows you to address specific concerns or offer personalized support.

Addressing Emotional and Practical Needs

- **Emotional Support:** Acknowledge that everyone will be experiencing a range of emotions, including grief, fear, anxiety, and anger. Offer emotional support and encourage family members to seek professional help if needed.

- **Practical Support:** Discuss practical matters related to caregiving responsibilities, financial planning, and funeral arrangements. Sharing these responsibilities can ease the burden on any one individual.

- **Delegation of Tasks:** Delegate specific tasks to family members based on their strengths and availability. This can help everyone feel involved and contribute to the caregiving effort.

Navigating Challenges and Difficult Conversations

- **Differing Opinions:** Disagreements about end-of-life care are common. Facilitate respectful discussions and try to find common ground. Focus on what's best for your loved one.

- **Family Dynamics:** Pre-existing family dynamics can influence communication patterns. Be mindful of these dynamics and try to create a supportive and inclusive environment.

- **Grief and Loss:** Grief can make communication challenging. Be patient and understanding with each other. Allow everyone to grieve in their own way.

Cultural Sensitivity

- **Respectful of Beliefs:** Be mindful of cultural and religious beliefs that may influence attitudes toward death and dying. Respect these beliefs and incorporate them into the care plan, as appropriate.

- **Open Dialogue:** Encourage open dialogue about cultural preferences and traditions related to end-of-life care.

Challenges to Communication and How to Overcome Them

- **Emotional Distress:** Grief, fear, and anxiety can make communication challenging. Acknowledge these emotions and seek support from others.

- **Cognitive Impairment:** If your loved one has cognitive impairment, communication may require patience, creativity, and nonverbal cues.

- **Differing Opinions:** Family members may have different opinions about end-of-life care. Facilitate respectful discussions and try to find common ground.

- **Cultural Differences:** Cultural beliefs and practices can influence communication styles and attitudes toward death and dying. Be sensitive to these differences and strive for understanding.

Effective communication is the cornerstone of compassionate end-of-life care. It allows individuals to express their wishes, receive the support they need, and experience their final days with dignity and peace. It also helps families navigate this difficult journey together, offering comfort, strength, and shared understanding.

Part 2

Practical Caregiving at End-of-Life

Chapter 5

Managing Physical Comfort

Pain

Pain management during end-of-life care is a critical aspect of ensuring comfort and dignity for individuals facing a life-limiting illness. It's a complex and often emotionally charged area, requiring caregivers to be informed, compassionate, and proactive in advocating for their loved ones.

Understanding Pain at the End of Life

Pain at the end of life can stem from various sources, including the underlying illness itself, related medical conditions, or even the treatments being administered. It can manifest as physical discomfort but also encompass emotional and spiritual suffering. Effective pain management requires a holistic approach, addressing all aspects of an individual's well-being.

- **Types of Pain:** Understanding the different types of pain can help caregivers communicate more effectively with the healthcare team. Pain can be categorized as:

- Nociceptive Pain: This is the most common type, caused by tissue damage and often described as aching, throbbing, or sharp.

- Neuropathic Pain: This results from damage to the nervous system and is often described as burning, tingling, shooting, or electric-like.

- Mixed Pain: Many individuals experience a combination of nociceptive and neuropathic pain.

- Pain Assessment: Accurately assessing pain is essential for effective management. However, at the end of life, individuals may have difficulty communicating their pain. Caregivers need to be observant and consider:

  - Verbal Cues: Listen carefully to what your loved one says about their pain, even if it's subtle or infrequent.

  - Nonverbal Cues: Pay close attention to nonverbal cues, such as facial expressions (grimacing, wincing), body language (restlessness, guarding), and changes in behavior (irritability, withdrawal).

  - Cognitive Impairment: If your loved one has cognitive impairment, pain assessment can be even more challenging. Rely heavily on nonverbal cues and input from the healthcare team.

The Role of the Caregiver in Pain Management

Caregivers play a vital role in ensuring effective pain management for their loved ones. Their responsibilities include:

- **Advocacy:** Caregivers are their loved one's primary advocates, ensuring their pain is adequately assessed and treated.

- **Communication:** Caregivers act as a bridge between their loved one and the healthcare team, communicating pain levels, changes in symptoms, and the effectiveness of treatments.

- **Observation:** Caregivers are often the first to notice changes in pain levels or new symptoms. Careful observation is crucial for timely intervention.

- **Administration of Medications:** Caregivers may be responsible for administering pain medications as prescribed by the healthcare team.

- **Comfort Measures:** Caregivers can provide various comfort measures to complement medical pain management.

Medical Approaches to Pain Management

The healthcare team will develop a personalized pain management plan based on the individual's specific needs and preferences. Common medical approaches include:

- **Pharmacological Interventions**

    - **Opioids:** These are potent pain medications commonly used for moderate to severe pain. Examples include morphine, oxycodone, and fentanyl. Opioids can be highly effective but also carry risks of side effects, such as constipation, nausea, and drowsiness.

    - **Non-opioid Analgesics:** These medications are used for mild to moderate pain. Examples include acetaminophen (Tylenol) and nonsteroidal anti-inflammatory drugs (NSAIDs) like ibuprofen (Advil, Motrin) and naproxen (Aleve). [1] NSAIDs should be used cautiously, especially in older adults, due to potential side effects.

    - **Adjuvant Medications:** These medications are used in combination with analgesics to enhance pain relief or manage specific types of pain, such as neuropathic pain. Examples include antidepressants, anticonvulsants, and corticosteroids.

- **Routes of Administration:** Pain medications can be administered in various ways, including:

  - **Oral:** This is the most common route, using pills, capsules, or liquids.

  - **Rectal:** This route may be used if the individual is unable to swallow.

  - **Transdermal:** Pain medication can be delivered through a patch applied to the skin.

  - **Subcutaneous or Intravenous:** These routes are used for more immediate pain relief or when other routes are not feasible.

Non-Medical Approaches to Pain Management

Complementary therapies can play an important role in managing pain and improving overall comfort. These approaches can be used alongside medical treatments.

- **Relaxation Techniques:** Deep breathing exercises, guided imagery, and meditation can help reduce muscle tension and promote relaxation, which can lessen pain perception.

- **Massage Therapy:** Gentle massage can help relieve muscle stiffness and improve circulation, which can ease pain.

- **Heat or Cold Therapy:** Applying heat or cold packs to the affected area can provide temporary pain relief.

- **Positioning and Repositioning:** Ensuring comfortable positioning and frequent repositioning can prevent pressure sores and reduce pain.

- **Distraction:** Engaging in enjoyable activities, such as listening to music, reading, or spending time with loved ones, can distract from pain and improve mood.

- **Acupuncture and Acupressure:** These traditional Chinese medicine techniques may help reduce certain types of pain.

- **Spiritual Support:** Addressing spiritual needs and finding meaning and purpose can contribute to overall well-being and pain management.

Managing Common Challenges in Pain Management

- **Constipation:** This is a common side effect of opioid medications. Caregivers should work with the healthcare team to implement strategies to prevent and manage constipation, such as increasing fluid intake, adding fiber to the diet, and using stool softeners or laxatives as needed.

- **Nausea and Vomiting:** Nausea and vomiting can also be side effects of some pain medications. The healthcare team can prescribe anti-nausea medications to manage these symptoms.

- **Drowsiness and Sedation:** Some pain medications can cause drowsiness or sedation. The healthcare team will adjust the dosage to balance pain relief with alertness.

- **Breakthrough Pain:** This refers to sudden flares of pain that occur despite regular pain medication. The healthcare team can prescribe additional medication to manage breakthrough pain.

- **Tolerance and Dependence:** With long-term use of opioid medications, tolerance may develop, requiring higher doses for the same level of pain relief. Physical dependence can also occur, meaning withdrawal symptoms may arise if the medication is stopped abruptly. The healthcare team will carefully monitor and manage these issues.

Ethical Considerations in End-of-Life Pain Management

- **The Principle of Double Effect:** This principle acknowledges that some treatments, such as pain medication, may have both intended (pain relief) and unintended (potential respiratory depression) effects. It supports the ethical use of medications to relieve suffering, even if they may hasten death, as long as the primary intent is to relieve pain and not to cause death.

- **Informed Consent:** Individuals have the right to make informed decisions about their pain management. Caregivers should ensure their loved ones have all the information they need to make choices that align with their values and preferences.

Communication with the Healthcare Team

Open and honest communication with the healthcare team is essential for effective pain management. Caregivers should:

- **Report Pain Levels:** Regularly report their loved one's pain levels to the healthcare team, including both verbal and nonverbal cues.

- **Describe Symptoms:** Provide detailed descriptions of any pain or other symptoms experienced.

- **Ask Questions:** Don't hesitate to ask questions about pain medications, side effects, or alternative therapies.

- **Share Concerns:** Express any concerns about pain management or treatment plans.

Pain management during end-of-life care is a complex and vital aspect of ensuring comfort and dignity. By understanding the different types of pain, utilizing both medical and non-medical approaches, and maintaining open communication with the healthcare team, caregivers can effectively advocate for their loved ones and help them experience a peaceful and comfortable end-of-life journey. Remember that the goal is not necessarily to eliminate all pain, but to manage it to a level that allows for meaningful connection and a sense of well-being in the time remaining.

Nausea

Nausea is a distressing symptom that can significantly impact quality of life during end-of-life care. It can be caused by a variety of factors, including the underlying illness, medications, or even emotional distress. Effectively managing nausea is a must for ensuring comfort and dignity in the final stages of life.

Understanding Nausea at the End of Life

Nausea, the feeling of unease and sickness in the stomach often accompanied by the urge to vomit, can be a complex symptom with multiple contributing factors at the end of life. It's essential to understand the potential causes to provide the most appropriate care.

- **Medication Side Effects:** Many medications commonly used in end-of-life care, particularly opioids for pain management, can cause nausea as a side effect.

- **Underlying Medical Conditions:** The terminal illness itself, such as cancer affecting the digestive system or advanced heart failure, can contribute to nausea.

- **Metabolic Imbalances:** Changes in the body's chemistry due to organ dysfunction can also trigger nausea.

- **Bowel Obstruction:** Blockages in the intestines can cause nausea and vomiting.

- **Constipation:** Severe constipation can contribute to feelings of nausea and bloating.

- **Dehydration:** Dehydration can exacerbate nausea.

- **Anxiety and Emotional Distress:** Psychological factors, such as anxiety, fear, and grief, can also manifest as nausea.

- **Tumor Involvement:** Tumors pressing on or affecting the digestive system can cause nausea.

- **Infections:** Certain infections can trigger nausea and vomiting.

The Caregiver's Role in Nausea Management

Caregivers are integral to effective nausea management at the end of life. Their responsibilities include:

- **Observation and Assessment:** Caregivers are often the first to notice signs of nausea. Careful observation of verbal and nonverbal cues is crucial.

- **Communication with the Healthcare Team:** Caregivers act as liaisons between their loved one and the healthcare team, relaying information about the frequency, severity, and potential triggers of nausea.

- **Administration of Medications:** Caregivers may be responsible for administering anti-nausea medications as prescribed by the healthcare team.

- **Implementation of Non-Pharmacological Strategies:** Caregivers can implement various non-medical strategies to complement medical interventions and enhance comfort.

- **Advocacy:** Caregivers advocate for their loved one's comfort and ensure their concerns about nausea are addressed by the healthcare team.

Medical Approaches to Nausea Management

The healthcare team will develop a personalized nausea management plan based on the individual's specific needs and the underlying causes of their nausea. Common medical approaches include:

- **Antiemetics:** These are medications specifically designed to relieve nausea and vomiting. Different types of antiemetics work in different ways, and the healthcare team will choose the most appropriate medication based on the cause of the nausea. Common examples include:

- **Ondansetron (Zofran):** Often used for nausea related to chemotherapy or surgery.

- **Metoclopramide (Reglan):** Can help with nausea related to slow stomach emptying.

- **Prochlorperazine (Compazine):** May be used for nausea related to medications or other causes.

- **Haloperidol (Haldol) or Lorazepam (Ativan):** May be used for nausea related to anxiety or delirium.

- **Route of Administration:** Antiemetics can be administered in various ways, including:

  - **Oral:** This is the most common route, using pills, capsules, or liquids.

  - **Rectal:** This route may be used if the individual is unable to swallow.

  - **Subcutaneous or Intravenous:** These routes are used for more immediate relief or when other routes are not feasible.

Non-Pharmacological Strategies for Nausea Relief

Complementary therapies can play a significant role in managing nausea and improving overall comfort. These approaches can be used alongside medical treatments:

- **Dietary Modifications**

    - **Small, Frequent Meals:** Eating small, frequent meals can be easier to tolerate than large meals.

    - **Bland Foods:** Bland, easily digestible foods, such as crackers, toast, or clear liquids, may be better tolerated when nauseated.

    - **Avoid Strong Odors:** Strong food odors can trigger nausea. Ensure the environment is well-ventilated and avoid cooking strong-smelling foods.

    - **Hydration:** Maintaining adequate hydration is crucial. Offer small sips of clear fluids, such as water, ginger ale, or clear broth. Ice chips or frozen juice pops can also be refreshing and hydrating.

- **Comfort Measures**

    - **Rest and Relaxation:** Resting in a comfortable position can help alleviate nausea. Encourage your loved one to lie down or recline in a quiet and peaceful environment.

○ **Cool Compress:** Applying a cool compress to the forehead or neck can provide some relief.

○ **Oral Care:** Maintaining good oral hygiene can help reduce nausea. Offer frequent mouth rinses with cool water or mouthwash.

○ **Deep Breathing:** Deep breathing exercises can help calm the nervous system and reduce nausea.

○ **Acupressure:** Applying pressure to specific acupressure points, such as the P6 point on the wrist, may help alleviate nausea.

○ **Ginger:** Ginger has natural anti-nausea properties. Ginger ale, ginger tea, or ginger candies may provide relief.

○ **Aromatherapy:** Certain essential oils, such as peppermint or ginger, may help reduce nausea when used in aromatherapy. However, it's important to use essential oils cautiously and ensure they are safe for use in end-of-life care. Consult with a healthcare professional or aromatherapist before using essential oils.

- **Environmental Modifications**

    - **Fresh Air:** Ensuring adequate ventilation and fresh air can help reduce nausea.

    - **Cool Room:** A cool room can be more comfortable for someone experiencing nausea.

    - **Quiet Environment:** Minimizing noise and distractions can help reduce nausea.

Managing Specific Challenges

- **Nausea and Vomiting:** If vomiting occurs, provide a basin and assist with oral care afterward. Keep the individual clean and comfortable.

- **Nausea and Medication Administration:** If nausea makes it difficult to take oral medications, talk to the healthcare team about alternative routes of administration, such as rectal, transdermal, or subcutaneous.

- **Persistent Nausea:** If nausea is persistent or severe, work closely with the healthcare team to adjust the medication regimen or explore other treatment options.

Communication with the Healthcare Team

Open and honest communication with the healthcare team is essential for effective nausea management. Caregivers should:

- **Report Nausea Episodes:** Inform the healthcare team about the frequency, severity, and any potential triggers of nausea.

- **Describe Symptoms:** Provide detailed descriptions of the nausea, including any associated symptoms, such as vomiting, dizziness, or abdominal discomfort.

- **Ask Questions:** Don't hesitate to ask questions about anti-nausea medications, side effects, or alternative therapies.

- **Share Concerns:** Express any concerns about nausea management or treatment plans.

Nausea during end-of-life care can significantly impact quality of life. By understanding the potential causes, utilizing both medical and non-pharmacological approaches, and maintaining open communication with the healthcare team, caregivers can effectively advocate for their loved ones and help them experience greater comfort and peace.

Shortness of Breath

Shortness of breath, also known as dyspnea, is a frightening and distressing symptom that can significantly impact quality of life during end-of-life care. The sensation of struggling to breathe can induce anxiety and fear, making it challenging for both the individual and their caregivers.

Understanding Shortness of Breath at the End of Life: A Multifaceted Challenge

Breathlessness at the end of life can arise from a variety of underlying causes, often interacting in complex ways. Understanding these potential contributors is essential for providing appropriate care:

- **Underlying Medical Conditions:** Many terminal illnesses, such as advanced lung disease (COPD, emphysema, lung cancer), heart failure, and neuromuscular diseases, directly affect respiratory function.

- **Fluid Buildup:** Fluid accumulation in the lungs (pulmonary edema or pleural effusion) can restrict lung expansion and contribute to breathlessness.

- **Anemia:** A low red blood cell count can reduce oxygen delivery to tissues, leading to shortness of breath.

- **Weakness of Respiratory Muscles:** The muscles responsible for breathing can weaken due to illness or immobility, making it harder to breathe deeply.

- **Anxiety and Emotional Distress:** Anxiety, fear, and emotional distress can exacerbate breathlessness, creating a vicious cycle.

- **Medication Side Effects:** Some medications can contribute to respiratory difficulties.

- **Positioning:** Certain positions can make breathing more difficult, especially for individuals with compromised lung function.

- **Environmental Factors:** Smoke, dust, allergens, or extreme temperatures can irritate the airways and worsen breathlessness.

The Caregiver's Vital Role: A Source of Comfort and Support

Caregivers are indispensable in managing breathlessness at the end of life. Their responsibilities include:

- **Observation and Assessment:** Caregivers are often the first to notice changes in breathing patterns or increased shortness of breath. They need to be observant and look for:

  - **Increased Respiratory Rate:** A rapid breathing rate can indicate difficulty breathing.

  - **Use of Accessory Muscles:** Observe if the individual is using muscles in the neck, chest, or abdomen to help them breathe.

- Nasal Flaring: Flaring of the nostrils can be a sign of respiratory distress.

- Chest Retractions: Observe if the chest is pulling inward between the ribs during inhalation.

- Changes in Skin Color: Bluish discoloration of the skin (cyanosis), especially around the lips and fingertips, can indicate low oxygen levels.

- Changes in Mental Status: Restlessness, anxiety, or confusion can be signs of respiratory distress.

- **Communication with the Healthcare Team:** Caregivers act as the primary communicators, relaying information about the frequency, severity, and potential triggers of breathlessness to the healthcare team.

- **Implementation of Comfort Measures:** Caregivers can implement a range of non-medical strategies to alleviate breathlessness and promote comfort.

- **Medication Administration:** Caregivers may be responsible for administering medications prescribed for breathlessness, such as oxygen therapy or nebulizers.

- **Emotional Support:** Providing reassurance, comfort, and a calm presence can significantly reduce anxiety and improve breathing.

Medical Approaches: Addressing the Underlying Cause

The healthcare team will develop a personalized plan to manage breathlessness based on the individual's specific needs and the underlying causes. Common medical approaches include:

- **Oxygen Therapy:** Supplemental oxygen can increase oxygen levels in the blood and ease breathlessness. Oxygen can be delivered through nasal cannulas, masks, or other devices.

- **Medications**

  - **Opioids:** Low doses of opioids, such as morphine, can help reduce the perception of breathlessness, even if they don't directly improve lung function.

  - **Bronchodilators:** These medications, often delivered via inhalers or nebulizers, relax the airways and make breathing easier. They are particularly helpful for individuals with asthma or COPD.

  - **Corticosteroids:** These medications can reduce inflammation in the airways and are sometimes used to treat breathlessness caused by certain lung conditions.

- o **Diuretics:** These medications help remove excess fluid from the body, which can be beneficial for individuals with fluid buildup in the lungs.

- **Other Interventions:**

  - o **Thoracentesis:** This procedure involves draining fluid from the space around the lungs (pleural effusion) to relieve pressure and improve breathing.

  - o **Paracentesis:** This procedure drains excess fluid from the abdomen, which can sometimes compress the lungs and cause breathlessness.

Non-Pharmacological Strategies: Enhancing Comfort and Control

Complementary therapies can play a central role in managing breathlessness and improving quality of life. These approaches can be used alongside medical treatments:

- **Positioning:**

  - o **Upright Position:** Sitting upright in a chair or propped up in bed with pillows can help expand the chest and make breathing easier.

  - o **Leaning Forward:** Leaning forward on a table or other support can also improve breathing mechanics.

- **Breathing Techniques**

  - **Pursed-Lip Breathing:** This technique involves breathing in through the nose and exhaling slowly through pursed lips. It can help control breathing and reduce shortness of breath.

  - **Diaphragmatic Breathing (Belly Breathing):** This technique involves breathing deeply from the diaphragm, which can improve lung capacity and reduce anxiety.

- **Relaxation Techniques**

  - **Deep Breathing Exercises:** Slow, deep breaths can help calm the nervous system and reduce anxiety associated with breathlessness.

  - **Guided Imagery:** Visualizing calming scenes can promote relaxation and reduce the perception of breathlessness.

  - **Meditation:** Regular meditation can help manage anxiety and improve overall well-being.

- **Cool Air:** A cool breeze from a fan directed towards the face can sometimes ease breathlessness.

- **Distraction:** Engaging in enjoyable activities, such as listening to music, reading, or spending time with loved ones, can distract from breathlessness and reduce anxiety.

- **Energy Conservation:** Pacing activities and avoiding strenuous exertion can help conserve energy and reduce shortness of breath.

- **Complementary Therapies:** Some individuals find relief from breathlessness through therapies like acupuncture or massage. However, it's important to consult with a healthcare professional before trying any new complementary therapies.

Managing Anxiety and Fear

Breathlessness can be very frightening, leading to anxiety and panic, which in turn can worsen the sensation of shortness of breath.

- **Reassurance:** Offer reassurance and a calm presence. Let your loved one know you are there for them and will do everything you can to help them breathe easier.

- **Calm Communication:** Speak calmly and gently. Avoid rushing or panicking, as this can increase anxiety.

- **Relaxation Techniques:** Guide your loved one through relaxation techniques, such as deep breathing or guided imagery.

- **Medications:** If anxiety is severe, the healthcare team may prescribe medications to help manage it.

Environmental Considerations

- **Fresh Air:** Ensure adequate ventilation and fresh air in the room.

- **Temperature:** A cool room can be more comfortable.

- **Minimize Irritants:** Avoid smoking, strong perfumes, or other irritants that can worsen breathlessness.

Communication with the Healthcare Team

Regular communication with the healthcare team is essential for effective management of breathlessness. Caregivers should:

- **Report Breathing Changes:** Inform the healthcare team about any changes in breathing patterns, increased shortness of breath, or new symptoms.

- **Describe Symptoms:** Provide detailed descriptions of the breathlessness, including when it occurs, what makes it better or worse, and any associated symptoms.

- **Ask Questions:** Don't hesitate to ask questions about medications, side effects, or alternative therapies.

- **Share Concerns:** Express any concerns about the management of breathlessness.

Managing shortness of breath during end-of-life care requires a comprehensive and compassionate approach. By understanding the potential causes, utilizing both medical and non-pharmacological strategies, and maintaining open communication with the healthcare team, caregivers will ensure their loved ones comfort.

Anxiety

Easing Anxiety During End-of-Life Care

Anxiety is a common and understandable experience during end-of-life. The uncertainty surrounding death, coupled with physical symptoms and emotional distress, can create a perfect storm for anxiety to arise.

Understanding Anxiety at the End of Life: A Complex Web of Factors

Anxiety at the end of life is rarely caused by a single factor. It's often a complex interplay of physical, emotional, and existential concerns. Understanding these contributing factors will help caregivers in providing holistic care:

- **Physical Symptoms:** Uncontrolled pain, shortness of breath, nausea, and other physical symptoms can trigger or exacerbate anxiety.

- **Fear of the Unknown:** The uncertainty surrounding death and what lies beyond can be a significant source of anxiety.

- **Emotional Distress:** Feelings of sadness, grief, regret, or unresolved conflicts can contribute to anxiety.

- **Spiritual Concerns:** Questions about the meaning of life, the afterlife, or unfinished spiritual business can lead to anxiety.

- **Changes in Cognitive Function:** Cognitive impairment due to illness or medications can make it difficult to process information and cope with emotions, leading to anxiety.

- **Environmental Factors:** A noisy, chaotic, or unfamiliar environment can increase anxiety.

- **Family Dynamics:** Tensions or unresolved issues within the family can contribute to anxiety for the dying individual.

The Caregiver's Role: A Source of Calm and Support

Caregivers are essential in recognizing and managing anxiety at the end of life. Their responsibilities include:

- **Observation and Assessment:** Caregivers are often the first to notice signs of anxiety in their loved ones. Look for:

    - **Verbal Cues:** Restlessness, irritability, difficulty concentrating, expressing fears or worries.

    - **Nonverbal Cues:** Facial expressions (frowning, grimacing, wide eyes), body language (fidgeting, pacing, trembling), changes in sleep patterns, changes in appetite.

- **Communication with the Healthcare Team** Share observations about your loved one's anxiety with the healthcare team, including specific symptoms, triggers, and any interventions that have been helpful.

- **Implementation of Comfort Measures:** Utilize non-pharmacological strategies to create a calm and supportive environment.

- **Emotional Support:** Provide reassurance, a listening ear, and a calming presence.

- **Advocacy:** Ensure your loved one's concerns about anxiety are addressed by the healthcare team and that they receive appropriate treatment.

Medical Approaches: Targeting the Source of Anxiety

The healthcare team will develop a personalized plan to manage anxiety based on the individual's specific needs and contributing factors. Common medical approaches include:

- **Medications**

    - **Anxiolytics:** These medications, such as lorazepam (Ativan) or alprazolam (Xanax), can help reduce anxiety symptoms.

    - **Antidepressants:** Certain antidepressants may be used to treat anxiety, particularly if depression is also present.

    - **Other Medications:** Medications used to manage other symptoms, such as pain or shortness of breath, can also have a positive impact on anxiety.

- **Route of Administration:** Medications for anxiety can be administered orally, rectally, subcutaneously, or intravenously, depending on the individual's needs and ability to take medications.

Non-Pharmacological Strategies

Complementary therapies can play a significant role in managing anxiety and promoting relaxation. These approaches can be used alongside medical treatments:

- **Creating a Calm Environment**

    - **Minimize Noise:** Reduce noise from televisions, radios, or conversations.

    - **Dim Lighting:** Soft, warm lighting can be more calming than bright lights.

    - **Comfortable Temperature:** Ensure the room is a comfortable temperature.

    - **Familiar Surroundings:** Surround your loved one with familiar objects, photos, or music that bring them comfort.

- **Relaxation Techniques**

    - **Deep Breathing:** Encourage slow, deep breaths to help calm the nervous system.

    - **Guided Imagery:** Guide your loved one through visualizations of peaceful scenes or positive memories.

    - **Progressive Muscle Relaxation:** This technique involves tensing and releasing different muscle groups to promote relaxation.

- o **Meditation:** Meditation can help calm the mind and reduce anxiety.

- **Touch:** Gentle touch, such as holding hands or stroking their arm, can provide comfort and reassurance.

- **Music Therapy:** Soothing music can have a calming effect and reduce anxiety.

- **Aromatherapy:** Certain scents, such as lavender or chamomile, may promote relaxation. However, use essential oils cautiously and consult with a healthcare professional or aromatherapist before using them, especially in end-of-life care.

- **Therapeutic Presence:** Simply being present with your loved one, offering a calm and supportive presence, can be incredibly comforting.

Addressing Specific Concerns

- **Fear of Dying:** Encourage open and honest conversations about fears and concerns related to death. Offer reassurance and explore spiritual or existential resources if desired.

- **Unfinished Business:** Help your loved one address any unfinished business or regrets they may have. This might involve facilitating conversations with loved ones, writing letters, or seeking spiritual guidance.

- **Spiritual Distress:** If spiritual concerns are contributing to anxiety, connect your loved one with a chaplain, spiritual advisor, or other spiritual support as desired.

Communication is Key: Sharing and Seeking Support

Open and consistent communication is essential for effective anxiety management. Caregivers should:

- **Report Anxiety Symptoms:** Inform the healthcare team about specific symptoms, frequency, and triggers of anxiety.

- **Share What Works:** Communicate any strategies or interventions that have been helpful in reducing anxiety.

- **Seek Guidance:** Don't hesitate to ask the healthcare team for advice and support in managing anxiety.

A Collaborative Approach to Comfort and Peace

Managing anxiety during end-of-life care requires a compassionate and collaborative approach involving the individual, their caregivers, and the healthcare team. By understanding the contributing factors, utilizing both medical and non-pharmacological strategies, and maintaining open communication, caregivers will ensure their loved ones have greater comfort, peace, and dignity in their final days or weeks.

Skin Changes

The skin, our body's largest organ, often reflects the changes occurring during the end-of-life journey. As bodily functions decline, the skin can become more fragile, susceptible to breakdown, and require specialized care.

Understanding Skin Changes at the End of Life: A Delicate Balance

Several factors contribute to skin changes as death approaches:

- **Decreased Circulation:** Reduced blood flow leads to less oxygen and nutrients reaching the skin, making it thinner, drier, and more vulnerable to injury.

- **Reduced Moisture:** Dehydration, decreased fluid intake, and changes in skin's ability to retain moisture contribute to dryness and cracking.

- **Loss of Subcutaneous Fat:** The layer of fat beneath the skin, which provides cushioning and insulation, diminishes, making the skin more susceptible to pressure sores.

- **Changes in Muscle Tone:** Muscle weakness can lead to decreased mobility, increasing the risk of pressure sores, especially over bony prominences.

- **Incontinence:** Exposure to urine and feces can irritate the skin, leading to rashes, breakdown, and infection.

- **Medical Conditions:** Underlying illnesses can directly affect skin integrity. For example, diabetes can impair wound healing, and edema (swelling) can put pressure on the skin.

- **Medications:** Some medications can have side effects that affect the skin, such as dryness, itching, or rashes.

Common Skin Changes at the End of Life

Caregivers should be aware of the following common skin changes:

- **Dryness and Cracking:** The skin may become dry, flaky, and prone to cracking, especially on the hands, feet, and elbows.

- **Thinning Skin:** The skin becomes thinner and more translucent, making blood vessels more visible and increasing vulnerability to tears and bruising.

- **Pressure Sores (Bedsores):** These develop when sustained pressure on the skin restricts blood flow, typically over bony prominences like the sacrum, hips, elbows, and heels. They can range from mild redness to deep wounds.

- **Skin Tears:** The fragile skin can tear easily with minimal friction or pressure.

- **Bruising:** Increased bruising can occur due to thinning skin and reduced clotting ability.

- **Rashes and Irritation:** Skin can become irritated due to incontinence, dryness, or reactions to products.

- **Infections:** Breaks in the skin can become infected, requiring prompt attention.

- **Edema (Swelling):** Fluid retention can cause swelling, particularly in the legs and ankles, putting pressure on the skin and increasing the risk of breakdown.

The Caregiver's Essential Role: Protecting and Preserving Skin Integrity

Caregivers responsibilities include:

- **Regular Skin Assessment:** Carefully inspect the skin daily, paying close attention to bony prominences, areas prone to pressure, and areas exposed to moisture. Look for any signs of redness, breakdown, or infection.

- **Hygiene and Cleansing:** Gentle cleansing is essential. Use warm water and a soft cloth or sponge. Avoid harsh soaps or scrubbing, which can irritate the skin.

- **Moisture Management:** Apply a moisturizing cream or lotion to dry skin to prevent cracking. Avoid products with perfumes or alcohol, which can further dry the skin.

- **Pressure Relief:** Implement strategies to relieve pressure on vulnerable areas:

    o **Frequent Repositioning:** Change the individual's position at least every two hours, or more frequently if needed.

    o **Specialized Mattresses and Cushions:** Use pressure-relieving mattresses, cushions, or overlays to distribute weight evenly.

    o **Pillows and Supports:** Use pillows to support the body and prevent pressure on bony prominences.

- **Incontinence Care:** Promptly clean and dry the skin after each episode of incontinence to prevent irritation and breakdown. Use barrier creams to protect the skin from urine and feces.

- **Wound Care:** If skin breakdown occurs, follow the healthcare team's instructions for wound care. Keep the wound clean and dressed appropriately.

- **Protection from Injury:** Take precautions to prevent skin tears and bruising. Dress the individual in soft, loose-fitting clothing. Be gentle when moving or transferring them.

- **Communication with the Healthcare Team:** Report any skin changes or concerns to the healthcare team promptly. They can provide guidance on appropriate care and treatment.

Specific Care Strategies for Common Skin Issues

- **Dry Skin:** Apply a fragrance-free, hypoallergenic moisturizer liberally after bathing and as needed throughout the day.

- **Pressure Sores:** Prevention is key. Frequent repositioning, pressure-relieving devices, and meticulous skin care are essential. If a pressure sore develops, follow the healthcare team's instructions for wound care.

- **Skin Tears:** Handle the skin gently. Cleanse the area with warm water and apply a dressing as directed by the healthcare team.

- **Incontinence-Associated Dermatitis:** Keep the skin clean and dry. Apply a barrier cream to protect the skin from urine and feces.

- **Infections:** Watch for signs of infection, such as redness, swelling, warmth, pain, or drainage. Report any suspected infection to the healthcare team immediately.

Creating a Comfortable and Supportive Environment

- **Soft Bedding and Clothing:** Use soft, breathable fabrics for bedding and clothing. Avoid rough seams or tags that can irritate the skin.

- **Temperature Control:** Maintain a comfortable room temperature. Extreme heat or cold can be drying and irritating to the skin.

- **Minimize Friction:** Be gentle when moving or transferring the individual. Use lifting aids or draw sheets to reduce friction on the skin.

Communication with the Healthcare Team

Regular communication with the healthcare team is crucial. Caregivers should:

- **Report Skin Changes:** Inform the healthcare team about any changes in the skin, including dryness, redness, breakdown, or signs of infection.

- **Describe Symptoms:** Provide detailed descriptions of any skin problems, including their location, size, and any associated symptoms.

- **Ask Questions:** Don't hesitate to ask questions about skin care products, wound care techniques, or other concerns.

Death Rattle

The death rattle, a gurgling or rattling sound produced by air passing through secretions in the upper respiratory tract of a dying person, can be a distressing experience for caregivers and family members. While it's a common occurrence in the final stages of life, understanding its causes, management strategies, and the emotional impact it can have will help the caregiver provide compassionate and informed care.

Understanding the Death Rattle: The Sound of Transition

The death rattle is not a sign of pain or distress for the dying individual. It's simply a mechanical sound caused by the movement of air over accumulated secretions in the throat and trachea. These secretions, often saliva, mucus, or fluids from the lungs, build up because the dying person's ability to swallow and clear their throat diminishes. It's important to remember that the dying person is usually unaware of the sound and is not suffering because of it.

Differentiating the Death Rattle from Other Respiratory Sounds

It's important to distinguish the death rattle from other respiratory sounds that may indicate distress:

- **Stertor:** This is a snoring-like sound caused by the tongue relaxing and obstructing the airway.

It can often be addressed by repositioning the individual.

- **Stridor:** This is a high-pitched whistling sound caused by an obstruction in the upper airway. It requires immediate medical attention.

- **Labored Breathing:** This involves visible effort to breathe, such as using accessory muscles (neck, chest, abdomen), nasal flaring, or chest retractions. It can indicate respiratory distress and should be assessed by the healthcare team.

The Caregiver's Role: Providing Comfort and Support

Witnessing the death rattle can be emotionally challenging for caregivers. Understanding its nature and having strategies to manage it can ease anxiety and allow for more focused care. The caregiver's role includes:

- **Understanding and Acceptance:** Recognizing that the death rattle is a natural part of the dying process can help caregivers cope with the emotional impact.

- **Communication with the Healthcare Team:** Caregivers should inform the healthcare team about the presence and nature of the death rattle.

- **Positioning and Comfort Measures:** Caregivers can implement several comfort

133

measures to minimize the sound and enhance the individual's comfort.

- **Emotional Support:** Providing emotional support to the dying person and their family is crucial during this time.

Management Strategies: Minimizing the Sound and Maximizing Comfort

The focus in managing the death rattle is on minimizing the sound and ensuring the individual's comfort, not necessarily eliminating the sound entirely. Here are some effective strategies:

- **Positioning**

  o **Lateral Position:** Turning the individual onto their side can help drain secretions and reduce the rattling sound.

  o **Elevated Head:** Raising the head of the bed or using pillows to support the upper body can also facilitate drainage.

- **Oral Care:** Gentle suctioning of the mouth and throat with a Yankauer suction catheter can remove secretions and temporarily reduce the sound. However, deep suctioning is generally not recommended as it can be uncomfortable and ineffective.

- **Medications**

- **Anticholinergics:** Medications like scopolamine or atropine can help dry up secretions and lessen the death rattle. These medications are typically administered via injection or transdermal patch. It's crucial to discuss the risks and benefits of these medications with the healthcare team.

- **Environmental Considerations**

  - **Quiet Environment:** Minimizing background noise can make the rattling sound less noticeable.

  - **Calm Atmosphere:** Creating a calm and peaceful environment can help reduce anxiety for both the dying person and their family.

Addressing Emotional Concerns: Supporting the Family

The death rattle can be particularly distressing for family members. Caregivers can play a vital role in providing emotional support:

- **Education:** Explain to family members that the death rattle is a common and natural part of the dying process and does not indicate pain or suffering.

- **Reassurance:** Offer reassurance and comfort. Let them know that you are doing everything possible to ensure their loved one is comfortable.

- **Emotional Support:** Provide a safe space for family members to express their feelings and concerns.

- **Spiritual Support:** If desired, connect the family with a chaplain or spiritual advisor.

Ethical Considerations: Balancing Comfort and Intervention

When considering interventions for the death rattle, it's essential to balance the potential benefits with the potential burdens for the dying individual.

- **Prioritize Comfort:** The primary goal is to ensure the individual's comfort and dignity.

- **Respect Wishes:** Honor the individual's wishes regarding end-of-life care, including their preferences for interventions.

- **Informed Consent:** Discuss the risks and benefits of any interventions with the healthcare team and the family, ensuring informed consent.

Communication with the Healthcare Team: A Collaborative Approach

Open and honest communication with the healthcare team is a must. Caregivers should:

- **Report the Death Rattle:** Inform the healthcare team about the presence and characteristics of the death rattle.

- **Discuss Management Options:** Discuss the various management strategies available, including positioning, suctioning, and medications.

- **Seek Guidance:** Ask the healthcare team for guidance on how to best manage the death rattle and provide comfort to the dying person.

Appetite and Thirst

As death approaches, significant changes occur in the body's systems, including a natural decrease in appetite and thirst. This is a common and often distressing experience for caregivers who may feel compelled to nourish their loved ones.

Understanding the Decline in Appetite and Thirst: A Natural Transition

The decrease in appetite and thirst during end-of-life care is primarily due to the body's slowing metabolism and reduced energy needs. As the body's systems begin to shut down, the need for food and fluids diminishes. This is a natural and expected part of the dying process, not a sign of neglect or a failure on the caregiver's part. Several factors contribute to this decline:

- **Reduced Metabolic Needs:** The body requires less energy as it begins to shut down. The need for calories and nutrients decreases significantly.

- **Decreased Digestive Function:** The digestive system slows down, making it harder to process food. This can lead to feelings of fullness, nausea, and constipation.

- **Weakened Muscles:** The muscles involved in chewing and swallowing may weaken, making eating and drinking more difficult and tiring.

- **Changes in Senses:** Taste and smell may become less acute, making food less appealing.

- **Underlying Medical Conditions:** The terminal illness itself can affect appetite and thirst.

- **Medications:** Some medications can cause nausea, loss of appetite, or a dry mouth, contributing to decreased intake.

- **Dehydration vs. Drying Mucous Membranes:** It's important to distinguish between true dehydration and the common symptom of drying mucous membranes in the mouth. While the dying person may appear dehydrated, aggressive hydration in the final stages can sometimes cause discomfort due to fluid overload.

The Caregiver's Role: Comfort, Not Coercion

Caregivers focus should shift from trying to force food and fluids to prioritizing comfort and addressing any distressing symptoms. The caregiver's role includes:

- **Understanding and Acceptance:** Recognizing that decreased appetite and thirst are a natural part of the dying process can help caregivers manage their own emotional responses.

- **Communication with the Healthcare Team:** Caregivers should inform the healthcare team about changes in eating and drinking patterns.

- **Offering Small Amounts of Preferred Foods:** If the individual expresses a desire for a particular food, offering a small portion can be a way to provide comfort and connection.

- **Providing Oral Care:** Keeping the mouth clean and moist is essential for comfort, even if the person is not eating or drinking much.

- **Managing Associated Symptoms:** Addressing any nausea, constipation, or other symptoms that may be affecting appetite and thirst.

- **Emotional Support:** Providing emotional support to both the dying person and their family members is essential during this time.

Strategies for Managing Decreased Appetite and Thirst

The focus should be on comfort and gentle encouragement, not force-feeding.

- **Offer Small Portions:** Small, frequent "meals" are often better tolerated than large meals. Offer small portions of preferred foods when the individual seems most alert and comfortable.

- **Respect Preferences:** Honor food and drink preferences, even if they seem unusual. The goal is to provide enjoyment and comfort, not necessarily a balanced diet.

- **Avoid Pressure:** Never force food or fluids. This can create distress and may lead to choking or aspiration (food or liquid entering the lungs).

- **Focus on Quality, Not Quantity:** The emphasis should be on offering small amounts of enjoyable food, not on meeting nutritional requirements.

- **Offer Soft Foods:** Soft, easily digestible foods, such as pureed fruits, yogurt, or pudding, may be easier to swallow.

- **Hydration Considerations:**

  - **Sips of Fluids:** Offer small sips of water, juice, or other preferred fluids if the individual is able to swallow.

- o **Ice Chips or Frozen Juice Pops:** These can be refreshing and help keep the mouth moist.

- o **Moistening the Mouth:** Use a moist sponge or cloth to keep the mouth and lips moist, even if the individual is not drinking much.

- o **Avoid Overhydration:** Aggressive hydration in the final stages can sometimes cause discomfort due to fluid overload. Discuss hydration needs with the healthcare team.

- **Oral Care**

  - o **Regular Cleaning:** Gently clean the mouth with a soft toothbrush or sponge several times a day.

  - o **Mouthwash:** Use a non-alcohol-based mouthwash to freshen the mouth.

  - o **Lip Balm:** Apply lip balm to prevent dryness and cracking.

- **Managing Associated Symptoms**

  - o **Nausea:** If nausea is present, work with the healthcare team to manage it with appropriate medications.

o **Constipation:** Address constipation with dietary modifications, increased fluid intake (if appropriate), or stool softeners as prescribed by the healthcare team.

o **Dry Mouth:** Use saliva substitutes or artificial saliva to keep the mouth moist.

Addressing Emotional Concerns

Family members may struggle with the decreased food and fluid intake of their loved one.

- **Provide Education:** Explain that this is a natural part of the dying process and not a sign of starvation.

- **Offer Support:** Provide emotional support to family members and reassure them that their loved one is not suffering because they are not eating or drinking much.

- **Focus on Comfort:** Shift the focus from food and fluids to providing comfort and companionship.

Communication with the Healthcare Team

- **Report Changes:** Inform the healthcare team about any significant changes in eating or drinking patterns.

- **Discuss Concerns:** Discuss any concerns about dehydration or other symptoms.

- **Seek Guidance:** Ask the healthcare team for guidance on how to best manage decreased appetite and thirst.

Embracing a Natural Transition

The decrease in appetite and thirst during end-of-life care is a natural and often unavoidable part of the dying process. By understanding the reasons behind this change, shifting the focus to comfort and gentle encouragement, and maintaining open communication with the healthcare team, caregivers can provide compassionate and supportive care during this sensitive time. Remember, the goal is not to prolong life artificially, but to maximize comfort and quality of life in the time remaining. Allowing the natural dying process to unfold, while providing comfort and love, is a profound act of caregiving.

Incontinence

Incontinence, the involuntary loss of bladder or bowel control, is a common and often emotionally distressing experience during end-of-life care. It can significantly impact a person's dignity and sense of self, and present unique challenges for caregivers.

Understanding Incontinence at the End of Life

Incontinence at the end of life can stem from a variety of factors, often interacting in complex ways:

- **Muscle Weakness:** The muscles controlling the bladder and bowel, including the pelvic floor muscles and sphincters, weaken as part of the body's natural slowing down process.

- **Nerve Damage:** Damage to the nerves that control bladder and bowel function, due to illness or neurological conditions, can contribute to incontinence.

- **Changes in Cognitive Function:** Cognitive impairment, such as dementia or delirium, can make it difficult for individuals to recognize the urge to go to the bathroom or to communicate their needs.

- **Medications:** Some medications can contribute to incontinence, either by affecting muscle control or increasing urine output.

- **Constipation:** Severe constipation can lead to bowel impaction and overflow incontinence.

- **Restricted Mobility:** Limited mobility can make it challenging to reach the toilet in time, leading to accidents.

- **Underlying Medical Conditions:** Conditions like diabetes, prostate enlargement, or urinary tract infections can also contribute to incontinence.

Types of Incontinence

Understanding the different types of incontinence can help caregivers better understand their loved one's experience and communicate more effectively with the healthcare team:

- **Urge Incontinence:** A sudden, strong urge to urinate followed by involuntary leakage.

- **Stress Incontinence:** Leakage of urine during physical activity, coughing, sneezing, or laughing.

- **Overflow Incontinence:** Frequent or constant dribbling of urine due to a full bladder that cannot empty completely.

- **Functional Incontinence:** Incontinence due to physical limitations or environmental barriers that prevent timely access to the toilet.

- **Mixed Incontinence:** A combination of different types of incontinence.

- **Bowel Incontinence:** Involuntary leakage of stool.

The Caregiver's Essential Role: Promoting Comfort and Dignity

Caregivers play a significant role in managing incontinence and supporting their loved ones through this challenging experience. Their responsibilities include:

- **Assessment and Observation:** Regularly assess for signs of incontinence, including wet clothing or bedding, skin irritation, or changes in behavior.

- **Hygiene and Skin Care:** Maintaining cleanliness and preventing skin breakdown are essential.

- **Continence Management:** Implementing strategies to manage incontinence, such as scheduled toileting, prompt assistance, and the use of absorbent products.

- **Emotional Support:** Providing compassionate and understanding support to minimize embarrassment and preserve dignity.

- **Communication with the Healthcare Team:** Informing the healthcare team about the type and frequency of incontinence episodes.

- **Advocacy:** Ensuring the individual's needs related to incontinence are addressed and that they receive appropriate care and support.

Strategies for Managing Incontinence

The approach to managing incontinence will depend on the type, severity, and underlying causes. Here are some effective strategies:

- **Scheduled Toileting:** Encourage regular trips to the toilet, even if there is no urge. Establish a toileting schedule based on the individual's usual pattern.

- **Prompt Assistance:** Provide prompt assistance to the toilet when needed. Ensure easy access to the bathroom or bedside commode.

- **Environmental Modifications:** Make the bathroom safe and accessible. Install grab bars, ensure adequate lighting, and remove any tripping hazards.

- **Absorbent Products:** Use absorbent pads, briefs, or diapers to manage incontinence and protect clothing and bedding. Choose products that are appropriate for the level of incontinence and comfortable for the individual.

- **Skin Care:**

    o **Gentle Cleansing:** Cleanse the skin gently with warm water and a soft cloth after each episode of incontinence. Avoid harsh soaps or scrubbing, which can irritate the skin.

    o **Barrier Creams:** Apply a barrier cream to protect the skin from urine and feces.

    o **Monitor for Skin Breakdown:** Regularly check for redness, rashes, or other signs of skin irritation.

- **Fluid Management:** Encourage adequate fluid intake to prevent dehydration, which can worsen constipation and incontinence. However, discuss fluid intake with the healthcare team, as some conditions may require fluid restriction.

- **Dietary Considerations:** A diet high in fiber can help prevent constipation and promote regular bowel movements.

- **Medications:** The healthcare team may prescribe medications to manage certain types of incontinence.

- **Pelvic Floor Exercises:** For individuals with stress incontinence, pelvic floor exercises (Kegel exercises) may be helpful in strengthening the pelvic floor muscles.

- **Catheters:** In some cases, a urinary catheter may be necessary to manage urinary incontinence. This is typically a decision made in consultation with the healthcare team.

- **Bowel Management Program:** For bowel incontinence, a bowel management program, including dietary modifications, regular toileting, and the use of stool softeners or laxatives as needed, may be recommended by the healthcare team.

Emotional and Psychological Support

Incontinence can be a source of significant embarrassment and shame, leading to social isolation and depression. The topic should be approached with dignity and respect in order to avoid embarrassing your loved one.

- **Respect and Dignity:** Treat the individual with respect and dignity. Acknowledge the emotional challenges associated with incontinence and offer reassurance.

- **Empathy and Understanding:** Show empathy and understanding. Let them know that they are not alone and that you are there to support them.

- **Positive Reinforcement:** Offer positive reinforcement and encouragement. Celebrate small successes in managing incontinence.

- **Privacy:** Ensure privacy during toileting and incontinence care.

- **Open Communication:** Encourage open communication about concerns and needs related to incontinence.

Communication with the Healthcare Team

- **Report Incontinence Episodes:** Inform the healthcare team about the frequency, type, and any associated symptoms of incontinence.

- **Discuss Management Options:** Discuss different management strategies and absorbent products with the healthcare team.

- **Seek Guidance:** Ask the healthcare team for guidance on how to best manage incontinence and provide emotional support.

Constipation

Constipation, infrequent or difficult bowel movements, is a common and often uncomfortable issue. It can significantly impact quality of life, contributing to discomfort, bloating, nausea, and even pain.

Understanding Constipation at the End of Life

Constipation at the end of life is rarely caused by a single factor. It's often a complex interplay of several contributing elements:

- **Slowed Digestive System:** The digestive tract's motility naturally slows down as the body's systems begin to shut down. This makes it harder for stool to move through the intestines.

- **Decreased Food and Fluid Intake:** Reduced food and fluid intake, common in the final stages of life, contributes to drier, harder stools that are more difficult to pass.

- **Medications:** Many medications used in end-of-life care, particularly opioids for pain management, can significantly contribute to constipation.

- **Inactivity:** Reduced physical activity and mobility can further slowdown the digestive system and exacerbate constipation.

- **Muscle Weakness:** Weakened abdominal and pelvic floor muscles can make it more difficult to have a bowel movement.

- **Underlying Medical Conditions:** Certain medical conditions, such as neurological disorders or bowel obstructions, can also contribute to constipation.

- **Dehydration:** Dehydration can lead to drier stools and make constipation worse.

The Caregiver's Essential Role: Promoting Comfort and Regularity

Responsibilities include:

- **Assessment and Monitoring:** Regularly monitor bowel movements, noting frequency, consistency, and any associated symptoms like straining, pain, or bloating.

- **Communication with the Healthcare Team:** Keep the healthcare team informed about bowel habits and any concerns about constipation.

- **Implementing Management Strategies:** Implement strategies to prevent and manage constipation, including dietary modifications, increased fluid intake (if appropriate), and medication administration.

- **Providing Comfort Measures:** Offer comfort measures to alleviate discomfort associated with constipation.

- **Emotional Support:** Provide emotional support and reassurance to the individual, who may feel embarrassed or distressed by constipation.

Strategies for Managing Constipation

The approach to managing constipation will depend on its severity and the individual's overall condition. Here are some effective strategies:

- **Dietary Modifications:**

  o **Increased Fiber (if appropriate):** If the individual is still eating, increasing fiber intake through fruits, vegetables, and whole grains can help bulk up stool and make it easier to pass. However, high-fiber intake may not be suitable in the very final stages of life or if there is a bowel obstruction. Discuss dietary changes with the healthcare team.

  o **Adequate Fluid Intake (if appropriate):** Ensure adequate fluid intake to keep stools soft. However, discuss appropriate fluid intake with the healthcare team, as some conditions may require fluid restriction. Small, frequent sips are often better tolerated than large amounts of fluid at once.

- **Regular Toileting Schedule:** Establish a regular toileting schedule, encouraging the individual to sit on the toilet or commode at consistent times each day, such as after meals.

- **Physical Activity (if possible):** Even gentle movement, if possible, can help stimulate the digestive system.

- **Stool Softeners:** Stool softeners, such as docusate sodium (Colace), can help soften stools and make them easier to pass.

- **Laxatives:** Laxatives, such as bisacodyl (Dulcolax) or senna (Senokot), can stimulate bowel movements. However, laxatives should be used cautiously and as directed by the healthcare team, as overuse can lead to dependence.

- **Suppositories or Enemas:** If other methods are ineffective, suppositories or enemas may be necessary to relieve constipation. These should be administered by a healthcare professional or a caregiver who has been properly trained.

- **Manual Disimpaction:** In cases of severe constipation or bowel impaction, manual disimpaction (removing stool manually) may be necessary. This should be performed by a healthcare professional.

Medications for Constipation

The healthcare team may prescribe specific medications to manage constipation, depending on the underlying cause and the individual's overall condition. These may include:

- **Stool Softeners:** Docusate sodium (Colace)
- **Osmotic Laxatives:** Polyethylene glycol (MiraLAX)
- **Stimulant Laxatives:** Bisacodyl (Dulcolax), Senna (Senokot)
- **Lubricant Laxatives:** Mineral oil
- **Chloride Channel Activators:** Lubiprostone (Amitiza) (used in specific situations)

Non-Pharmacological Approaches

Several non-pharmacological approaches can complement medical interventions:

- **Abdominal Massage:** Gentle abdominal massage can help stimulate bowel movements.

- **Warm Compress:** Applying a warm compress to the abdomen can be soothing and may help relieve discomfort.

- **Privacy and Comfort:** Ensure privacy and a comfortable environment for toileting.

Addressing Emotional Concerns

Constipation can be a source of embarrassment and discomfort, affecting the individual's emotional well-being. Caregivers should:

- **Offer Reassurance:** Reassure the individual that constipation is a common issue and that you are there to help.

- **Maintain Dignity:** Treat the individual with respect and dignity. Ensure privacy during toileting and bowel care.

- **Open Communication:** Encourage open communication about bowel habits and any concerns.

Communication with the Healthcare Team

- **Report Bowel Movements:** Inform the healthcare team about the frequency and consistency of bowel movements.

- **Discuss Concerns:** Discuss any concerns about constipation or related symptoms.

Seek Guidance: Ask the healthcare team for guidance on how to best manage constipation and provide comfort.

Chapter 6

Providing Personal Care

Providing personal care during end-of-life care is a deeply intimate and meaningful way to show love and support. It's about more than just physical hygiene; it's about preserving dignity, fostering comfort, and maintaining connection during a vulnerable time.

Understanding the Importance of Personal Care

Personal care at the end of life goes beyond basic hygiene. It encompasses:

- **Physical Comfort:** Keeping the individual clean, comfortable, and free from pain or discomfort related to their physical needs.

- **Emotional Well-being:** Maintaining a sense of dignity and self-worth through respectful and compassionate care.

- **Connection and Intimacy:** Using personal care as an opportunity to connect with your loved one through gentle touch, conversation, and shared moments.

Bathing/Skin Care

- **Frequency:** Bathing frequency will likely decrease as energy levels decline. Focus on keeping the individual clean and comfortable, even if a full bath isn't always possible.

- **Sponge Baths:** Sponge baths are often the most comfortable option. Use warm water, a soft cloth, and gentle soap. Pay attention to skin folds and areas prone to pressure sores.

- **Skin Care:** Apply moisturizer to dry skin, especially after washing. Be gentle and avoid rubbing vigorously. Pay attention to areas prone to pressure sores (bony prominences).

- **Pressure Sore Prevention:** Frequent repositioning (at least every two hours), pressure-relieving mattresses and cushions, and meticulous skin care are crucial for preventing pressure sores.

As a person's strength and energy decline, traditional bathing methods may become too strenuous or uncomfortable. The goal shifts from a thorough cleansing to maintaining hygiene and promoting well-being.

Understanding the Changing Needs

- **Decreased Energy:** Individuals at the end of life often have very little energy. Traditional showers or baths can be exhausting and potentially unsafe.

- **Skin Fragility:** Skin becomes thinner and more fragile, making it more susceptible to tearing and bruising. Harsh soaps and vigorous scrubbing should be avoided.

- **Reduced Mobility:** Limited mobility can make it difficult to get in and out of the shower or tub.

- **Temperature Sensitivity:** Sensitivity to temperature changes may increase. Pay close attention to water temperature and room temperature.

Prioritizing Comfort and Dignity

- **Respect Preferences:** Always involve the individual in decisions about bathing. Respect their preferences regarding frequency, timing, and method.

- **Privacy:** Ensure privacy during bathing. Close doors or use screens to shield the individual from view.

- **Warmth:** Keep the room warm and comfortable to prevent chills.

- **Gentle Approach:** Use a gentle, compassionate approach. Explain what you are doing before you do it.

- **Minimizing Movement:** Keep movements slow and deliberate to avoid causing pain or discomfort.

Alternatives to Traditional Bathing

- **Sponge Baths:** Sponge baths are often the most comfortable and practical option for individuals at the end of life.

    o **Prepare:** Gather all necessary supplies beforehand: warm water, soft cloths or sponges, gentle soap, a towel, and a basin.

    o **Procedure:** Begin with the face and then wash the rest of the body, paying attention to skin folds and areas prone to pressure sores. Rinse with clean water and pat the skin dry gently.

- **Towel Baths:** Towel baths use pre-moistened cloths to cleanse the skin. They are a quick and convenient option, especially if the individual has limited mobility.

- **No-Rinse Cleansers:** No-rinse cleansers are designed to cleanse the skin without the need for water. They can be helpful for specific areas or for quick cleanups.

Specific Areas of Focus

- **Face:** Wash the face gently with warm water and a soft cloth. Pay attention to the eyes, nose, and mouth.

- **Mouth Care:** Oral care is essential, even if the individual is not eating. Use a soft-bristled toothbrush or foam swab to clean the mouth, tongue, and gums. Keep the mouth moist with frequent sips of water (if possible), ice chips, or mouthwash.

- **Perineal Care:** Keep the perineal area clean and dry, especially after episodes of incontinence. Use warm water and a soft cloth. Apply a barrier cream if necessary to protect the skin from irritation.

- **Hair Care:** Regularly brush the hair to prevent tangles. Consider dry shampoo or no-rinse shampoo if traditional shampooing is difficult.

- **Nail Care:** Keep nails trimmed to prevent them from becoming too long or sharp.

Managing Common Challenges

- **Skin Breakdown:** If skin breakdown occurs, consult with the healthcare team for guidance on wound care.

- **Pressure Sores:** Prevent pressure sores by frequent repositioning (at least every two hours), using pressure-relieving mattresses and cushions, and meticulously caring for the skin.

- **Incontinence:** If incontinence is an issue, use absorbent pads, briefs, or diapers. Change them frequently and cleanse the skin thoroughly after each episode.

- **Pain:** If the individual is experiencing pain, ensure that pain medication is administered before bathing to minimize discomfort.

Working with the Healthcare Team

- **Communication:** Maintain open communication with the healthcare team about any concerns or challenges related to bathing.

- **Guidance:** Seek guidance from nurses or other healthcare professionals on specific techniques or products that may be helpful.

- **Collaboration:** Work collaboratively with the healthcare team to develop a personal care plan that meets the individual's needs and preferences.

Key Considerations

- **Adaptability:** Be prepared to adapt bathing routines as the individual's condition changes.

- **Focus on Comfort:** The primary goal is to ensure comfort and dignity.

- **Respect Wishes:** Honor the individual's wishes and preferences regarding bathing.

- **Emotional Connection:** Use bathing as an opportunity to connect with your loved one and express your love and support.

Oral Care

- o **Regular Cleaning:** Even if the individual isn't eating much, oral care is essential. Use a soft-bristled toothbrush or a foam swab to clean the mouth, tongue, and gums.

- o **Moisturizing:** Keep the mouth moist with frequent sips of water (if possible), ice chips, or mouthwash. Lip balm can prevent dry, cracked lips.

- o **Denture Care:** If the individual wears dentures, clean them regularly and ensure they fit comfortably.

Even if a person is no longer eating or drinking, maintaining oral hygiene remains essential.

Why Oral Care Matters at the End of Life

- **Comfort:** A clean and moist mouth contributes significantly to overall comfort. Dry mouth, sores, or infections can cause significant discomfort.

- **Dignity:** Maintaining oral hygiene helps preserve a sense of dignity and well-being.

- **Prevention of Complications:** Poor oral care can lead to infections, sores, and discomfort, further impacting quality of life.

- **Communication:** Keeping the mouth clean and moist can make communication easier, even if it's just a few words or sips of water.

Common Oral Care Challenges at End of Life

- **Dry Mouth (Xerostomia):** This is a very common issue due to decreased saliva production, medications, and dehydration.

- **Sores and Infections:** Mouth sores (stomatitis) can develop due to illness, medications, or poor oral hygiene. Thrush (oral candidiasis), a yeast infection, is also common.

- **Difficulty Swallowing:** Weakened muscles can make swallowing difficult, increasing the risk of aspiration (food or liquid entering the lungs).

- **Decreased Awareness:** Cognitive decline can make it difficult for individuals to communicate their oral care needs or participate in their care.

Essential Oral Care Supplies

- **Soft-bristled toothbrush or foam swabs:** Choose a gentle option to avoid irritating sensitive tissues.

- **Non-alcohol-based mouthwash:** Alcohol can dry out the mouth further.

- **Moisturizing mouth spray or gel:** These products can help relieve dry mouth.

- **Lip balm:** Prevents dry, cracked lips.

- **Small cup of water or ice chips:** For rinsing or moistening the mouth.

- **Towel or cloth:** For wiping the mouth and chin.

- **Gloves:** For infection control.

Oral Care Routine

1. **Hand Hygiene:** Wash your hands thoroughly before and after providing oral care.

2. **Assessment:** Gently examine the mouth for any sores, redness, or signs of infection.

3. **Cleaning:**

   o **Brushing:** If the individual can tolerate it, gently brush their teeth and gums with a soft-bristled toothbrush and a small amount of toothpaste.

- ○ **Foam Swabs:** If brushing is too difficult, use foam swabs to clean the mouth. Moisten the swab with water or mouthwash and gently clean the teeth, gums, and tongue.

4. **Rinsing:** Offer small sips of water or ice chips for rinsing if the individual is able to swallow. If not, use a moist cloth or sponge to gently wipe the mouth.

5. **Moisturizing:** Apply moisturizing mouth spray or gel to relieve dryness.

6. **Lip Care:** Apply lip balm to prevent dry, cracked lips.

7. **Denture Care (if applicable):** Clean dentures daily and ensure they fit comfortably. Remove dentures at night to allow the gums to rest.

Managing Specific Oral Care Challenges

- **Dry Mouth:**

  - ○ Frequent moisturizing with sprays, gels, or artificial saliva.

  - ○ Offer small sips of water or ice chips (if able to swallow).

  - ○ Avoid sugary drinks, which can worsen dryness.

- o Use a humidifier in the room.

- **Sores and Infections:**

  - o Report any sores or signs of infection to the healthcare team.

  - o Follow their recommendations for treatment, which may include medicated mouthwash or ointments.

  - o Avoid spicy or acidic foods that can irritate sores.

- **Difficulty Swallowing:**

  - o Offer small sips of fluids between meals.

  - o Thicken liquids if necessary to make them easier to swallow.

  - o Position the individual upright during oral care to minimize the risk of aspiration.

- **Decreased Awareness:**

  - o Provide oral care regularly, even if the individual doesn't ask for it.

  - o Be gentle and reassuring.

  - o Talk to the individual during oral care, even if they are not responsive.

Communication and Collaboration

- **Healthcare Team:** Communicate regularly with the healthcare team about any oral care concerns or changes you observe. They can provide guidance and recommend appropriate treatments.

- **Family Members:** Share information about the individual's oral care needs and preferences with other family members involved in their care.

Key Considerations for End-of-Life Oral Care

- **Adaptability:** Be prepared to adapt the oral care routine as the individual's condition changes.

- **Prioritize Comfort:** The primary goal is to ensure comfort and prevent discomfort.

- **Respect Wishes:** Honor the individual's wishes and preferences regarding oral care.

- **Gentle and Consistent Care:** Consistent and gentle oral care is crucial for maintaining comfort and preventing complications.

Hair Care

- **Gentle Brushing:** Regularly brush the hair to prevent tangles and keep it looking neat.

- o **Shampooing:** Shampooing may be less frequent. Consider dry shampoo or using a no-rinse shampoo if traditional shampooing is difficult.

- o **Shaving:** If the individual is accustomed to shaving, continue to do so if they wish and it is comfortable.

Hair care during end-of-life care is about more than just aesthetics; it's a way to maintain dignity, comfort, and connection. As a person's energy levels decrease and their condition changes, hair care routines may need to be adapted. The goal is to keep the hair clean, comfortable, and looking as well as possible without causing undue stress or discomfort.

Understanding the Importance of Hair Care

- **Dignity:** Maintaining hair care can help a person feel more like themselves and preserve a sense of dignity during a vulnerable time.

- **Comfort:** Tangled or matted hair can be uncomfortable and even painful. Regular hair care can prevent this.

- **Connection:** Hair care can be a gentle and intimate way to connect with your loved one and show your care.

Challenges in End-of-Life Hair Care

- **Decreased Energy:** The individual may have very little energy for hair care.

- **Reduced Mobility:** Washing and styling hair can be difficult if the person has limited mobility.

- **Skin Sensitivity:** The scalp may become more sensitive, requiring gentle products and techniques.

- **Medication Side Effects:** Some medications can affect hair growth or texture.

Essential Hair Care Supplies

- **Soft-bristled brush:** Choose a brush that is gentle on the scalp.

- **Wide-toothed comb:** Helps detangle hair without pulling.

- **Gentle shampoo (optional):** Choose a mild, fragrance-free shampoo. Dry shampoo is a good alternative.

- **Conditioner (optional):** Can help manage tangles and dryness.

- **Towel:** For drying hair.

- **Basin or sink (if using water):** For washing hair.

- **Dry shampoo (optional):** A good alternative to traditional shampoo.

- **No-rinse shampoo (optional):** Another alternative to traditional shampoo.

- **Hair ties or clips:** For styling hair.

Hair Care Routine

Respect Preferences: Always involve the individual in decisions about their hair care. Ask them what they prefer and respect their choices.

Gentle Brushing: Regularly brush the hair to prevent tangles and remove loose hair. Be gentle and avoid pulling.

Washing (if desired and able):

- **Traditional Shampooing (if possible):** If the individual is able and prefers a traditional shampoo, assist them as needed. Use warm water and a gentle shampoo. Be mindful of their comfort and energy levels.

- **Dry Shampoo:** Dry shampoo is a great option for cleaning hair without water. Simply spray it on the hair, massage it in, and brush it out.

- ○ **No-Rinse Shampoo:** No-rinse shampoo is another waterless option. Apply it to the hair, massage it in, and towel dry.

Conditioning (if desired): Apply conditioner to the hair if it is dry or tangled.

Drying: Gently towel dry the hair. Avoid using a hair dryer unless it is on a cool setting and the individual tolerates it well.

Styling: Style the hair in a way that is comfortable and familiar to the individual. This could be as simple as combing it or putting it up in a ponytail or bun.

Managing Specific Hair Care Challenges

- **Tangled Hair:** Use a wide-toothed comb and gently work through tangles, starting at the ends and working your way up. Consider using a detangling spray.

- **Matted Hair:** If the hair is severely matted, it may be necessary to carefully cut out the mats. Consult with a healthcare professional or hairdresser for assistance.

- **Dry Hair:** Use a moisturizing conditioner or hair oil to add moisture and prevent breakage.

- **Oily Hair:** If the hair becomes oily, dry shampoo can be used between washes.

- **Hair Loss:** Hair loss can be a side effect of some medications or illnesses. Be gentle when brushing and styling the hair.

Creating a Comfortable and Dignified Experience

- **Privacy:** Ensure privacy during hair care.

- **Warmth:** Keep the room warm to prevent chills.

- **Pace:** Allow plenty of time for hair care. Don't rush.

- **Comfort:** Prioritize comfort. If something is uncomfortable, stop and try a different approach.

- **Emotional Support:** Provide emotional support and reassurance. Let the individual know that you are there for them and that you care.

Nail Care

- **Trimming:** Keep nails trimmed to prevent them from becoming too long or sharp, which could cause injury.

○ **Moisturizing:** Apply lotion to the hands and feet, paying attention to the cuticles.

Nail care is an often overlooked aspect of personal care, but it can significantly contribute to comfort, dignity, and overall well-being. Keeping nails clean, trimmed, and moisturized can prevent discomfort, reduce the risk of injury, and promote a sense of self-worth during a vulnerable time.

Why Nail Care Matters at the End of Life

- **Comfort:** Long or sharp nails can scratch or irritate the skin, causing discomfort. Keeping nails trimmed prevents this.

- **Hygiene:** Clean nails help prevent the spread of germs and reduce the risk of infection, especially important when skin integrity may be compromised.

- **Dignity:** Well-maintained nails contribute to a sense of overall well-being and can help a person feel more like themselves.

- **Prevention of Injury:** Long nails can snag on clothing or bedding, potentially leading to tears in fragile skin.

Challenges in End-of-Life Nail Care

- **Decreased Mobility:** It can be difficult for individuals with limited mobility to care for their own nails.

- **Skin Fragility:** The skin around the nails may be thin and easily injured.

- **Circulatory Issues:** Poor circulation can affect nail growth and health.

- **Cognitive Decline:** Individuals with cognitive impairment may not be aware of their nail care needs or be able to participate in the process.

Essential Nail Care Supplies

- **Nail clippers or scissors:** Choose tools that are easy to grip and maneuver.

- **Nail file (emery board):** For smoothing rough edges.

- **Hand lotion or cuticle oil:** To moisturize and prevent dryness.

- **Basin of warm water (optional):** For soaking hands and feet.

- **Towel:** For drying hands and feet.

- **Gloves (optional):** For infection control.

Nail Care Routine

Respect Preferences: Always involve the individual in decisions about their nail care. Ask them if they would like their nails trimmed and how they prefer them shaped.

Hand Hygiene: Wash your hands thoroughly before and after providing nail care.

Assessment: Gently examine the nails and surrounding skin for any signs of infection, such as redness, swelling, or drainage.

Soaking (optional): If the individual is comfortable and it is feasible, soak their hands and feet in a basin of warm water for a few minutes to soften the nails and cuticles.

Trimming:

- **Fingernails:** Trim fingernails straight across, following the natural shape of the finger. Avoid cutting into the corners of the nails, as this can increase the risk of ingrown nails.

- **Toenails:** Trim toenails straight across as well. It's especially important to avoid cutting into the corners of toenails, as this can easily lead to ingrown nails, especially for individuals with diabetes or circulatory issues.

- **Diabetes:** Do not use nail clippers on a person with diabetes. Nails should be filed only. Even the smallest wound can be difficult to heal so you don't want to risk clipping the skin.

Filing: Use a nail file to smooth any rough edges and prevent snags. File in one direction only, rather than sawing back and forth.

Moisturizing: Apply hand lotion or cuticle oil to moisturize the nails and surrounding skin.

Cleaning: Gently clean under the nails with a soft brush or cotton swab.

Managing Specific Nail Care Challenges

- **Thickened Nails:** If the nails are thick or difficult to cut, consult with a podiatrist or other healthcare professional for assistance.

- **Ingrown Nails:** If an ingrown nail develops, consult with a healthcare professional for treatment. Do not attempt to treat it yourself.

- **Brittle Nails:** Brittle nails can be prone to breakage. Keep them trimmed short and moisturized.

- **Fungal Infections:** If you notice any signs of a fungal infection, such as discoloration, thickening, or crumbling nails, consult with a healthcare professional for diagnosis and treatment.

Creating a Comfortable and Dignified Experience

- **Privacy:** Ensure privacy during nail care.

- **Warmth:** Keep the room warm to prevent chills.

- **Positioning:** Position the individual comfortably, ensuring easy access to their hands and feet.

- **Pace:** Allow plenty of time for nail care. Don't rush.

- **Gentle Touch:** Use gentle touch and be mindful of any areas of pain or sensitivity.

- **Emotional Support:** Provide emotional support and reassurance. Let the individual know that you are there for them and that you care.

Working with the Healthcare Team

- **Communication:** Maintain open communication with the healthcare team about any concerns or challenges related to nail care.

- **Guidance:** Seek guidance from nurses or other healthcare professionals on specific techniques or products that may be helpful.

Toileting and Incontinence Care

○ **Scheduled Toileting:** Encourage regular trips to the bathroom or bedside commode, even if the individual doesn't feel the urge.

○ **Incontinence Management:** If incontinence is an issue, use absorbent pads, briefs, or adult diapers. Change them frequently to prevent skin irritation.

○ **Skin Care:** Cleanse the skin thoroughly after each episode of incontinence and apply a barrier cream to protect the skin.

Establishing a toileting schedule can be immensely helpful for both the individual and their caregivers. While it might seem rigid at first, a well-implemented schedule can significantly improve quality of care.

Benefits for the Individual

- **Reduced Incontinence Episodes:** Regular toileting can help prevent accidents by anticipating the need to go. This is especially helpful for individuals with urge incontinence (a sudden, strong urge) or functional incontinence (difficulty reaching the toilet).

- **Improved Comfort:** A regular bowel and bladder routine can minimize discomfort associated with a full bladder or bowel, such as bloating, urgency, or pain.

- **Preserved Dignity:** Reducing incontinent episodes helps maintain a sense of dignity and control, which is particularly important during a vulnerable time.

- **Reduced Anxiety:** Knowing when to expect toileting can reduce anxiety and worry about having an accident.

- **Better Sleep:** A regular toileting schedule, especially if it includes nighttime toileting, can minimize nighttime disruptions and improve sleep quality.

- **Increased Awareness of Bodily Functions:** A schedule can help the individual become more aware of their body's signals, even if they are subtle.

Benefits for Caregivers

- **Reduced Caregiver Burden:** A toileting schedule can make caregiving more manageable by creating a predictable routine. It can reduce the frequency of unexpected cleanups and clothing changes.

- **Improved Skin Care:** Regular toileting and prompt cleaning after incontinent episodes can help prevent skin breakdown and pressure sores.

- **Enhanced Comfort for the Individual:** Knowing their loved one is comfortable and clean can provide peace of mind for caregivers.

- **Better Management of Supplies:** A schedule can help caregivers anticipate the need for incontinence supplies, such as pads or briefs, and ensure they are readily available.

- **More Time for Meaningful Interactions:** By streamlining toileting routines, caregivers can have more time for meaningful interactions, emotional support, and other important aspects of end-of-life care.

How to Implement a Toileting Schedule

Observe and Document: Start by observing the individual's current toileting patterns. Note the frequency of urination and bowel movements, any accidents, and any related symptoms. Keep a record for a few days to identify patterns.

Establish a Routine: Based on the observed patterns, create a toileting schedule. This might involve toileting every 2-4 hours during the day and perhaps once or twice at night.

Offer Toileting Assistance: Assist the individual to the toilet or bedside commode at the scheduled times, even if they don't express the urge to go.

Provide Privacy and Comfort: Ensure privacy and a comfortable environment for toileting.

Offer Fluids Regularly: Encourage regular fluid intake (if appropriate and as directed by the healthcare team) to help maintain regular bowel movements and prevent dehydration, which can worsen constipation and incontinence.

Dietary Considerations: If the individual is still eating, a balanced diet with adequate fiber (if appropriate and as directed by the healthcare team) can help promote regular bowel movements.

Incontinence Products: If incontinence is an issue, use appropriate absorbent products, such as pads or briefs, and change them promptly after each episode.

Skin Care: Pay close attention to skin care, especially in areas prone to irritation from urine or stool. Cleanse the skin gently after each episode and apply a barrier cream if necessary.

Medication Management: Discuss any medications that may be affecting bowel or bladder function with the healthcare team. They may be able to adjust medications or recommend other interventions.

Flexibility and Adaptation: Be prepared to adjust the schedule as needed. End-of-life care involves constant changes, and the toileting schedule may need to be modified based on the individual's condition and preferences.

Communication with the Healthcare Team: Keep the healthcare team informed about the individual's toileting habits and any concerns you may have. They can offer guidance and recommend additional strategies.

Important Considerations

- **Respect and Dignity:** Approach toileting assistance with respect and sensitivity. Maintain the individual's privacy and dignity at all times.

- **Individual Preferences:** Involve the individual in the toileting schedule as much as possible. Respect their preferences and allow them to participate in the process to the extent they are able.

- **Comfort and Safety:** Prioritize comfort and safety during toileting. Ensure the bathroom or bedside commode is easily accessible and safe to use.

- **Focus on Quality of Life:** The goal of a toileting schedule is to improve quality of life, not to impose a rigid routine. Be flexible and adapt the schedule as needed to meet the individual's changing needs and preferences.

Choosing the right incontinence products

Types of Incontinence Products

- **Adult Diapers/Briefs:** These offer the most comprehensive protection, suitable for moderate to heavy incontinence, both urinary and bowel. They come in various absorbencies and styles, including tab-style (with adhesive tabs) and pull-up styles.

  - **Tab-style briefs:** Best for individuals with limited mobility or those who require assistance with changes.

  - **Pull-up underwear:** Suitable for more mobile individuals who can manage changes independently.

- **Pads/Liners:** These are smaller and more discreet than briefs, ideal for light to moderate urinary incontinence. They can be worn inside regular underwear or with special holders.

- **Underwear/Protective Underwear:** These look and feel like regular underwear but have built-in absorbent layers. They are suitable for light to moderate incontinence and offer more discretion than briefs.

- **Bed Pads/Chux:** These are placed on beds, chairs, or other surfaces to protect them from accidents. They are helpful for managing incontinence overnight or for individuals with limited mobility.

Key Features to Consider

- **Absorbency:** Choose products with an absorbency level that matches the individual's needs. Consider overnight protection for nighttime use.

- **Skin Health:** Look for products with a breathable outer layer to promote airflow and prevent skin irritation. Some products also contain skin-soothing ingredients.

- **Odor Control:** Many incontinent products have odor-neutralizing properties to help maintain discretion.

- **Comfort and Fit:** Choose products that fit comfortably and securely to prevent leaks and skin irritation. Consider features like elastic leg gathers and adjustable closures.

- **Ease of Use:** Opt for products that are easy to put on and take off, especially for individuals with limited mobility or caregivers who are assisting with changes.

- **Disposability:** Most incontinent products are disposable, but some reusable options are available. Consider the environmental impact and cost when making your choice.

Product Recommendations

- **NorthShore GoSupreme Overnight Incontinence Underwear:** These pull-up style briefs offer excellent overnight protection and a snug fit to prevent leaks. They are a popular choice for heavy incontinence.

- **Tranquility Premium Overnight Disposable Absorbent Underwear:** These are highly absorbent overnight pull-on diapers that provide superior protection for a restful sleep.

- **Tena Overnight Super Underwear:** These pull-on underwear are designed for overnight use and offer good absorbency and a comfortable fit.

- **Abena Abri-Form Premium Brief:** These tab-style briefs are known for their high quality and absorbency, making them suitable for heavy incontinence.

- **CVS Health Protective Pads Ultimate Absorbency:** These pads offer discreet protection for light to moderate urinary incontinence and are readily available at most drugstores.

Tips for Choosing the Right Products

- **Start with a Sample Pack:** Many companies offer sample packs that allow you to try different products before committing to a larger purchase.

- **Consider Individual Needs:** The best product will depend on the individual's specific needs, including the level of incontinence, mobility, and personal preferences.

- **Consult with Healthcare Professionals:** Talk to the healthcare team for advice on choosing the most appropriate incontinent products. They can assess the individual's needs and recommend specific brands or types of products.

- **Read Reviews:** Online reviews can provide valuable insights into the pros and cons of different products.

- **Look for Promotions:** Many companies offer discounts or promotions on incontinent products.

Considerations for End-of-Life Care

- **Skin Integrity:** Prioritize products that are gentle on the skin and help prevent skin breakdown.

- **Ease of Changes:** Choose products that are easy to put on and take off, especially for individuals with limited mobility or those who require assistance with changes.

- **Comfort:** Opt for products that are comfortable and do not cause irritation or discomfort.

- **Dignity:** Select products that help maintain the individual's sense of dignity and self-worth.

By carefully considering these factors and exploring the available options, caregivers can choose the best incontinent products to meet their loved one's needs and ensure their comfort and well-being.

Dressing

- o **Comfortable Clothing:** Dress the individual in comfortable, loose-fitting clothing that is easy to put on and take off.

- o **Layering:** Layer clothing to adjust to temperature changes.

- o **Personal Preferences:** Respect the individual's preferences regarding clothing.

Clothing Considerations

The goal is to choose garments that are gentle on the skin, easy to put on and take off, and allow for easy access for medical care and personal care.

Key Clothing Considerations

- **Comfort:** This is paramount. Choose soft, breathable fabrics like cotton, bamboo, or blends that are gentle on sensitive skin. Avoid rough textures, itchy materials (like wool), or anything that could cause pressure or irritation.

- **Ease of Dressing/Undressing:** Look for clothing with easy closures like snaps, Velcro, or large buttons. Avoid complicated fastenings. Garments that open completely, like robes or gowns, can be especially helpful for individuals with limited mobility.

- **Accessibility for Medical Care:** Choose clothing that allows easy access for medical examinations, wound care, or IV lines. Loose-fitting garments or those with openings can be beneficial.

- **Dignity:** While comfort is key, it's also important to consider the individual's sense of dignity. Choose clothing that makes them feel comfortable and as "dressed" as they would like to be. Even if they are mostly in bed, a clean, comfortable top can make a difference.

- **Temperature Regulation:** Individuals at the end of life may have difficulty regulating their body temperature. Layering clothing allows for easy adjustments if they become too hot or too cold.

- **Personal Preferences:** Respect the individual's clothing preferences as much as possible. If they have favorite items, try to incorporate them into their wardrobe.

- **Practicality:** Consider the practicality of caring for the clothing. Choose garments that are easy to wash and dry.

Types of Clothing to Consider

- **Loose-fitting gowns or robes:** These are comfortable, easy to put on and take off, and allow for easy access for medical care.

- **Adaptive clothing:** This specialized clothing is designed for individuals with limited mobility or other physical challenges. It often features easy closures and openings.

- **Soft, comfortable pajamas:** Pajamas can be worn day or night and offer comfort and ease of movement.

- **T-shirts and sweatpants:** These are comfortable and easy to care for. Choose soft fabrics and loose fits.

- **Socks:** Soft, seamless socks can help keep feet warm and comfortable. Avoid tight elastic bands that could restrict circulation.

- **Underwear:** Choose soft, breathable underwear, even if incontinent products are being used.

Specific Clothing Tips

- **Avoid tight clothing:** Tight clothing can restrict circulation and cause discomfort, especially for individuals with edema or other physical changes.

- **Choose seamless garments:** Seams can rub against sensitive skin and cause irritation.

- **Opt for front-opening garments:** These are easier to put on and take off, especially for individuals with limited mobility.

- **Consider the environment:** If the individual is in a hospital or care facility, they may prefer clothing that is easy for staff to manage.

- **Label clothing:** Label all clothing with the individual's name to prevent loss or mix-ups, especially in shared care settings.

- **Keep a few favorite outfits readily available:** Having a few preferred outfits on hand can make dressing easier and more comfortable.

Remember

- **Focus on comfort:** Prioritize comfort above all else.

- **Respect preferences:** Honor the individual's clothing preferences as much as possible.

- **Be flexible:** Be prepared to adapt clothing choices as the individual's condition changes.

- **Gentle care:** Handle clothing gently when dressing and undressing to avoid causing injury or discomfort.

Creating a Comfortable and Dignified Experience

- **Respect and Dignity:** Treat the individual with respect and dignity throughout the personal care process.

- **Privacy:** Ensure privacy during personal care activities.

- **Communication:** Communicate clearly and gently. Explain what you are doing before you do it.

- **Inclusion:** Involve the individual in the process as much as possible. Allow them to make choices and express their preferences.

- **Gentle Touch:** Use gentle touch and be mindful of any areas of pain or sensitivity.

- **Pace:** Allow plenty of time for personal care activities. Don't rush.

- **Comfort:** Prioritize comfort. If something is uncomfortable, stop and try a different approach.

- **Emotional Support:** Provide emotional support and reassurance. Let the individual know that you are there for them and that you care.

Providing personal care is a profound act of love and service. It's a time to cherish precious moments and provide compassionate care with gentleness and understanding.

Chapter 7

Creating a Comfortable Environment

Creating a comfortable environment fosters a space that is physically and emotionally supportive, allowing for meaningful moments and a peaceful transition.

Why Creating a Comfortable Environment is Important

Creating a comfortable environment is profoundly important for several interconnected reasons, all centered around maximizing quality of life during a very sensitive and vulnerable time. It's not just about physical comfort, but about holistic well-being.

Physical Comfort and Symptom Management

- **Pain Management:** A comfortable environment can contribute to better pain management. Things like proper positioning, comfortable bedding, and a calm atmosphere can help reduce pain perception and allow pain medication to be more effective.

- **Symptom Relief:** Many end-of-life symptoms, such as shortness of breath, nausea, or restlessness, can be exacerbated by environmental factors. A calm, cool, and well-ventilated space can offer relief.

- **Preventing Complications:** A clean and comfortable environment, along with proper bedding and positioning, is crucial for preventing pressure sores, skin breakdown, and other complications that can cause further discomfort.

Emotional and Psychological Well-being

- **Reducing Anxiety and Fear:** A peaceful and familiar environment can significantly reduce anxiety and fear, which are common emotions at the end of life. The presence of familiar objects, loved ones, and a sense of calm can provide reassurance and comfort.

- **Promoting Relaxation and Peace:** A comfortable environment fosters relaxation and a sense of peace, allowing the individual to focus on meaningful moments and connections with loved ones.

- **Preserving Dignity:** Maintaining a clean, comfortable, and respectful environment helps preserve the individual's dignity during a time when they may feel particularly vulnerable.

- **Supporting Emotional Processing:** A safe and supportive environment allows for emotional processing and expression. It provides a space where the individual can express their feelings, fears, and hopes without judgment.

Spiritual Well-being

- **Facilitating Reflection:** A quiet and peaceful environment allows for introspection and spiritual reflection. It provides the space for the individual to connect with their inner self and address any spiritual needs.

- **Supporting Rituals:** A comfortable environment can facilitate spiritual practices and rituals that are important to the individual, such as prayer, meditation, or spending time with religious objects.

Family and Loved Ones

- **Providing a Space for Connection:** A comfortable environment allows family and loved ones to gather and spend precious time with the dying individual. It fosters meaningful connections and shared moments.

- **Easing Caregiver Burden:** A well-organized and comfortable environment can make caregiving tasks easier and less stressful, allowing caregivers to focus on providing emotional support and spending quality time with their loved one.

- **Creating Positive Memories:** The environment in which someone dies can leave a lasting impression on family members. Creating a peaceful and comfortable space can help create more positive memories of the final days or weeks.

Overall Quality of Life

Ultimately, creating a comfortable environment during end-of-life care is about maximizing the individual's quality of life during a time when it matters most. It's about minimizing suffering, promoting peace, and allowing for meaningful connections with loved ones. It's about honoring the individual's dignity and respecting their wishes for how they want to spend their final days. It's a vital aspect of providing compassionate and holistic end-of-life care.

Key Elements of a Comfortable Environment

Physical Comfort:

- **Temperature:** Maintain a comfortable room temperature. Individuals at the end of life may have difficulty regulating their body temperature, so it's essential to avoid extremes of hot or cold. Layering blankets can help them adjust as needed.

- **Lighting:** Opt for soft, warm lighting. Avoid harsh or bright lights, which can be irritating. Natural light is often preferred, but ensure it's not too glaring.

- **Noise:** Minimize noise levels. A quiet and peaceful environment can promote relaxation and reduce anxiety. Limit loud conversations, television, and other distractions. Soft, calming music may be welcomed by some.

- **Air Quality:** Ensure good ventilation and fresh air. Avoid strong odors, perfumes, or air fresheners, which can be irritating or trigger nausea.

- **Cleanliness:** Maintain a clean and tidy environment. Regular cleaning can help prevent odors and create a more pleasant atmosphere.

- **Comfortable Bedding:** Use soft, comfortable bedding, such as cotton sheets and blankets. Pressure-relieving mattresses or overlays can be helpful for individuals with limited mobility or those at risk for pressure sores.

- **Positioning:** Ensure comfortable positioning in bed or a recliner. Use pillows to support the body and relieve pressure points. Frequent repositioning is essential to prevent discomfort and skin breakdown.

Emotional and Psychological Comfort

- **Presence:** Simply being present with the individual can be incredibly comforting. Your presence conveys love, support, and companionship.

- **Emotional Support:** Offer emotional support and reassurance. Listen attentively to their concerns and fears. Avoid giving unsolicited advice or trying to "fix" their emotions.

- **Respect and Dignity:** Treat the individual with respect and dignity throughout the end-of-life journey. Honor their wishes and preferences as much as possible.

- **Meaningful Connections:** Encourage meaningful connections with family and friends. Facilitate visits, phone calls, or video chats as desired.

- **Spiritual Support:** If the individual is religious or spiritual, provide access to spiritual resources, such as clergy, spiritual advisors, or sacred texts.

- **Memory Sharing:** Sharing memories and stories can be a comforting and meaningful way to connect with the individual.

- **Creating a Peaceful Atmosphere:** A calm and peaceful atmosphere can help reduce anxiety and promote relaxation. This might involve playing soft music, lighting candles (if allowed and safe), or simply spending quiet time together.

Personal Touches

- **Familiar Objects:** Surround the individual with familiar and comforting objects, such as photos, artwork, or personal items. These can provide a sense of connection to their life and loved ones.

- **Personal Care Items:** Ensure access to personal care items, such as toiletries, favorite blankets, or clothing. Maintaining personal routines can contribute to a sense of normalcy and dignity.

- **Music:** If the individual enjoys music, play their favorite songs or create a playlist of calming music.

- **Nature:** If possible, bring nature indoors. A vase of flowers or a view of a garden can be uplifting.

Music and sound can play a profound role in comforting a person. They can evoke memories, reduce anxiety, ease pain, and provide a sense of connection and peace during a vulnerable time. Here's how:

The Power of Music

- **Emotional Connection:** Music has a unique ability to tap into emotions and memories. Familiar songs can evoke powerful feelings of joy, love, comfort, or nostalgia, providing a sense of connection to the past.

- **Anxiety and Stress Reduction:** Calming music can help reduce anxiety and stress, promoting relaxation and a sense of peace. It can distract from physical discomfort and create a more tranquil atmosphere.

- **Pain Management:** Studies have shown that music can have a positive impact on pain perception. It can act as a distraction and may even trigger the release of endorphins, the body's natural painkillers.

- **Spiritual Connection:** For some individuals, music can be a pathway to spiritual connection. Hymns, religious music, or songs with spiritual significance can provide comfort and solace.

- **Sense of Control:** Allowing the individual to choose the music they listen to can give them a sense of control during a time when they may feel a loss of control over many aspects of their life.

- **Communication and Connection:** Music can be a form of nonverbal communication, especially when verbal communication becomes difficult. Sharing music with loved ones can be a way to connect and express love and appreciation.

The Role of Sound

- **Nature Sounds:** Sounds of nature, such as ocean waves, rain, or birdsong, can be calming and soothing. They can create a peaceful and tranquil atmosphere.

- **White Noise:** White noise can help mask disturbing sounds and create a more peaceful environment. This can be particularly helpful in a hospital or care facility.

- **Familiar Sounds:** The sounds of loved ones' voices, even if they are just chatting or reading aloud, can be comforting and reassuring.

- **Silence:** Sometimes, silence can be just as powerful as music or sound. Periods of quiet can allow for reflection, introspection, and a sense of peace.

How to Use Music and Sound Effectively

- **Personalized Playlists:** Create personalized playlists of the individual's favorite music. Include songs that have special meaning to them or that evoke positive memories.

- **Variety:** Offer a variety of music and sounds to choose from. Preferences may change from day to day or even hour to hour.

- **Volume:** Keep the volume at a comfortable level. Loud music can be overwhelming or irritating.

- **Timing:** Offer music and sound at times when the individual seems most receptive. Be mindful of their energy levels and avoid playing music when they are trying to rest.

- **Shared Listening:** Share music with the individual and their loved ones. This can be a beautiful way to connect and spend quality time together.

- **Live Music:** If possible, consider having live music played for the individual. The presence of a musician can be a special and meaningful experience.

- **Respect Preferences:** Always respect the individual's preferences regarding music and sound. If they don't want to listen to music or if they prefer silence, honor their wishes.

- **Observe and Adapt:** Pay attention to the individual's responses to different types of music and sound. Adjust the playlist and volume as needed.

Important Considerations

- **Cognitive Decline:** Even if the individual is no longer verbally communicative, they may still be able to respond to music and sound. Pay attention to nonverbal cues, such as facial expressions or body movements.

- **Hearing Impairment:** If the individual has hearing impairment, consider using headphones or a portable speaker placed close to their ear.

- **Cultural Considerations:** Be mindful of cultural preferences regarding music and sound. What is considered calming in one culture may be different in another.

Creating a comfortable environment is an ongoing process that requires flexibility and sensitivity. By paying attention to the physical, emotional, and spiritual needs of the individual, caregivers can create a space that promotes peace, comfort, and meaningful connection during the final stages of life.

Chapter 8

Nutritional Considerations

Providing nutrition and hydration during end-of-life care is a complex and sensitive issue, often raising ethical dilemmas for caregivers and healthcare providers. It's essential to understand the available options, their potential benefits and burdens, and the ethical considerations involved in making these decisions.

Options for Providing Nutrition and Hydration

- **Oral Intake:** This is the most natural and preferred method. Encourage the individual to eat and drink as desired, offering small portions of preferred foods and fluids. However, as death approaches, the desire for food and fluids naturally diminishes.

- **Enteral Nutrition:** This involves delivering nutrients directly to the stomach or small intestine through a feeding tube.

  This may be considered when the individual is unable to swallow or consume enough nutrition orally, but their digestive system is still functioning.

- ○ **Nasogastric Tube (NG tube):** A tube inserted through the nose into the stomach.

- ○ **Percutaneous Endoscopic Gastrostomy (PEG tube):** A tube inserted through the abdomen into the stomach.

- ○ **Jejunostomy Tube (J tube):** A tube inserted into the jejunum (part of the small intestine).

- **Parenteral Nutrition:** This involves delivering nutrients directly into the bloodstream through an intravenous (IV) line. This may be considered when the digestive system is not functioning properly or when other methods are not feasible.

- **Parenteral Hydration:** This involves administering fluids directly into the bloodstream through an IV line to prevent dehydration.

Ethical Considerations

- **Autonomy:** Respecting the individual's autonomy and their right to make decisions about their own care is paramount. This includes their right to refuse or withdraw any form of treatment, including nutrition and hydration.

- **Beneficence:** Acting in the best interests of the individual is a core ethical principle. This involves weighing the potential benefits and burdens of providing nutrition and hydration.

- **Non-maleficence:** Avoiding harm is another essential ethical principle. It's crucial to consider the potential risks and burdens of artificial nutrition and hydration, such as infection, aspiration, fluid overload, and discomfort.

- **Justice:** Ensuring fair and equitable access to care is also important. This includes providing adequate information and support to individuals and their families to make informed decisions about nutrition and hydration.

Factors to Consider

- **Individual's Wishes:** The individual's wishes and preferences regarding nutrition and hydration should be honored. Advance directives, such as a living will or durable power of attorney for healthcare, can provide guidance in this regard.

- **Medical Condition:** The individual's medical condition, prognosis, and goals of care should be taken into account. In some cases, artificial nutrition and hydration may prolong the dying process without providing any significant benefit.

- **Potential Benefits and Burdens:** The potential benefits and burdens of providing nutrition and hydration should be carefully considered. While these interventions can provide nourishment and prevent dehydration, they can also lead to complications and discomfort.

- **Quality of Life:** The impact of nutrition and hydration on the individual's overall quality of life should be assessed. In some cases, artificial nutrition and hydration may detract from the individual's comfort and ability to engage in meaningful activities.

- **Cultural and Spiritual Beliefs:** Cultural and spiritual beliefs may influence decisions about nutrition and hydration at the end of life. These beliefs should be respected and taken into account.

Making Decisions

Decisions about providing nutrition and hydration during end-of-life care should be made collaboratively between the individual, their family, and the healthcare team. Open and honest communication is essential.

- **Provide Information:** The healthcare team should provide accurate and comprehensive information about the options available, their potential benefits and burdens, and the ethical considerations involved.

- **Facilitate Discussion:** The healthcare team can facilitate discussions between the individual and their family to help them explore their values, beliefs, and preferences.

- **Support Decision-Making:** The healthcare team should support the individual and their family in making informed decisions that are consistent with their values and goals of care.

Food Options

The best food options will depend on the individual's specific circumstances, preferences, and ability to swallow.

General Guidelines:

- **Small Portions:** Offer small, frequent "meals" rather than large meals. The individual may only be able to eat very small amounts at a time.

- **Respect Preferences:** Honor food and drink preferences, even if they seem unusual. The goal is to provide enjoyment and comfort, not necessarily a balanced diet.

- **Avoid Pressure:** Never force food or fluids. This can create distress and may lead to choking or aspiration (food or liquid entering the lungs).

- **Focus on Quality, Not Quantity:** The emphasis should be on offering small amounts of enjoyable food, not on meeting nutritional requirements.

- **Soft and Easily Digestible Foods:** These are generally easier to swallow and digest.

- **Hydration Considerations:** Offer small sips of water, juice, or other preferred fluids if the individual is able to swallow. Ice chips or frozen juice pops can also be refreshing and help keep the mouth moist. Be mindful of potential fluid overload, especially if there are concerns about kidney function. Discuss hydration needs with the healthcare team.

Food Options to Consider

- **Soft and Pureed Foods:**

  - **Yogurt:** Smooth and easy to swallow, provides some protein and calcium.

  - **Applesauce:** A classic choice, easy to digest and soothing.

  - **Pureed Fruits and Vegetables:** Offer a variety of flavors and some nutrients. Consider sweet potato, banana, avocado, or pureed berries.

  - **Baby Food:** Convenient and readily available in various flavors.

  - **Smoothies:** A good way to combine fruits, yogurt, or even protein powder (if appropriate and desired).

- o **Broth-based Soups:** Provide hydration and some nutrients.

- **Other Soft Foods:**

  - o **Mashed Potatoes:** Easy to swallow and can be flavored to the individual's liking.

  - o **Scrambled Eggs:** A good source of protein and relatively easy to eat.

  - o **Pudding or Custard:** A sweet treat that is easy to swallow.

  - o **Ice Cream or Sherbet:** Cool and refreshing, can be soothing for a sore mouth.

- **Fluids:**

  - o **Water:** Offer small sips frequently.
  - o **Juice:** Diluted juice may be more palatable.
  - o **Broth:** A good source of electrolytes and fluids.
  - o **Ice Chips:** Helpful for keeping the mouth moist.
  - o **Frozen Juice Pops:** Refreshing and hydrating.

Foods to Avoid:

- **Dry or Crunchy Foods:** These can be difficult to chew and swallow.

- **Sticky or Clumpy Foods:** These can be hard to swallow and may increase the risk of choking.

- **Highly Acidic or Spicy Foods:** These can irritate a sore mouth or cause discomfort.

- **Large Portions:** These can be overwhelming and may lead to nausea or vomiting.

Important Considerations

- **Oral Care:** Even if the individual is eating very little, oral care is essential. Regular mouth cleaning with a soft toothbrush or foam swab and moisturizing the lips can improve comfort.

- **Medication Side Effects:** Be aware that some medications can affect taste and appetite. Discuss any concerns with the healthcare team.

- **Changes in Taste:** Taste buds can change as death approaches. Foods that were once enjoyed may no longer be appealing. Be flexible and willing to try different options.

- **Listen to the Individual:** Pay close attention to the individual's cues and preferences. If they don't want to eat or drink, don't force them.

- **Focus on Enjoyment:** The goal is to provide pleasure and comfort, not to meet specific nutritional goals. If the individual enjoys a particular food, offer it, even if it's not considered "nutritious."

- **Hydration:** While maintaining hydration is important, avoid overhydration, which can cause discomfort. Discuss appropriate fluid intake with the healthcare team.

Remember

- **This is a natural process:** Changes in appetite and eating habits are a normal part of the dying process.

- **Comfort is key:** Prioritize comfort and quality of life over trying to force food or fluids.

- **Respect wishes:** Honor the individual's wishes and preferences regarding food and drink.

- **Seek support:** Don't hesitate to ask for help from the healthcare team, family members, or friends.

Considerations of Artificial Nutrition

While artificial nutrition (enteral or parenteral) can be a valuable intervention in certain situations, it's crucial to be aware of the potential complications, especially during end-of-life care. The risks and burdens often outweigh the benefits in the final stages of life, and it's important to weigh these factors carefully with the healthcare team and the individual (if possible).

Complications of Enteral Nutrition (Tube Feeding)

- **Aspiration Pneumonia:** This is a serious complication where food or fluids are inhaled into the lungs, leading to pneumonia. It's a particular risk for individuals with swallowing difficulties, reduced consciousness, or reflux.

- **Infection:** Infections can occur at the insertion site of the feeding tube (skin infection) or within the digestive system.

- **Tube-Related Issues:**

    o **Tube blockage:** The feeding tube can become blocked, requiring replacement or intervention.

    o **Tube dislodgement:** The tube can be accidentally pulled out, requiring reinsertion.

    o **Skin irritation/pressure sores:** The tube can irritate the skin around the insertion site, leading to pressure sores, especially with long-term use.

- **Gastrointestinal Issues:**

    - **Nausea and vomiting:** Tube feeding can cause nausea, vomiting, or diarrhea.

    - **Abdominal distention and cramping:** The volume or rate of feeding can cause discomfort.

    - **Constipation or diarrhea:** Changes in bowel habits are common.

- **Metabolic Imbalances:** Imbalances in electrolytes or blood sugar can occur, requiring careful monitoring and management.

- **Psychological Distress:** The presence of a feeding tube can be distressing for some individuals, affecting their body image or sense of well-being.

Complications of Parenteral Nutrition (IV Feeding)

- **Infection:** Infections of the central line catheter (the IV line placed for TPN) are a significant risk and can be life-threatening.

- **Blood Clots:** Blood clots can form in the vein where the catheter is inserted.

- **Metabolic Imbalances:** TPN can cause significant imbalances in electrolytes, blood sugar, and other nutrients, requiring frequent monitoring and adjustment.

- **Liver Problems:** Long-term TPN can lead to liver damage or dysfunction.

- **Fluid Overload:** TPN can cause fluid overload, leading to swelling, respiratory distress, and heart failure, particularly in individuals with compromised heart or kidney function.

- **Pneumothorax:** This is a collapsed lung that can occur during the insertion of the central line catheter.

- **Psychological Distress:** The presence of an IV line can be distressing for some individuals.

General Considerations for Artificial Nutrition at End of Life

- **Ethical Concerns:** As mentioned previously, the ethical principles of autonomy, beneficence, non-maleficence, and justice must be carefully considered. The potential burdens of artificial nutrition may outweigh the benefits in the final stages of life, especially when the individual's prognosis is very limited.

- **Quality of Life vs. Prolonging Dying:** Artificial nutrition may prolong the dying process without significantly improving the quality of life. It's important to consider whether the intervention aligns with the individual's goals of care.

- **Comfort vs. Nutrition:** In the final stages of life, the focus often shifts from providing nutrition to ensuring comfort. Aggressive nutritional support may cause more discomfort than benefit.

- **Dehydration vs. Drying Mucous Membranes:** It's crucial to differentiate between true dehydration and the common symptom of drying mucous membranes in the mouth. While the dying person may appear dehydrated, aggressive hydration in the final stages can sometimes cause discomfort due to fluid overload. Small sips of fluids, ice chips, or moistening the mouth with a sponge may be more appropriate and comfortable.

- **Informed Decision-Making:** Decisions about artificial nutrition should be made collaboratively between the individual (if possible), their family, and the healthcare team. The individual's wishes and preferences should be honored.

It's essential to have open and honest conversations with the healthcare team about the potential risks and benefits of artificial nutrition in the context of the individual's overall condition, prognosis, and goals of care. The decision should be based on what is in the best interest of the individual and what aligns with their values and wishes for their end-of-life care.

Important Considerations

- **Artificial nutrition and hydration are medical interventions:** Like any other medical intervention, they should be evaluated based on their potential benefits and burdens in the context of the individual's overall condition and goals of care.

- **There is no moral obligation to provide artificial nutrition and hydration in all cases:** The decision to provide or withhold artificial nutrition and hydration should be based on a careful assessment of the individual's specific circumstances and their wishes.

- **Comfort is paramount:** The primary goal of end-of-life care is to ensure comfort and quality of life. If artificial nutrition and hydration are causing discomfort or detracting from the individual's overall well-being, they may be reconsidered or withdrawn.

Decisions about nutrition and hydration at the end of life can be challenging. By understanding the available options, considering the ethical implications, and engaging in open communication with the healthcare team, individuals and their families can make informed choices that align with their values and promote a peaceful and dignified end-of-life experience.

Chapter 9

Medication Management

Medication administration during end-of-life care can be complex, requiring careful consideration of dosage adjustments, route changes, and side effect management. It's vital for caregivers to work closely with the healthcare team to ensure safe and effective medication management.

Dosage Adjustments

- **Changes in Metabolism:** As the body's systems slow down, metabolism can be affected, leading to slower drug processing. This means medications may stay in the system longer, increasing the risk of side effects. Dosage adjustments may be necessary, especially for medications with a narrow therapeutic window.

- **Organ Function:** Declining liver and kidney function can impact drug clearance. These organs play a crucial role in eliminating medications from the body. Impaired function can lead to drug accumulation and toxicity, requiring dosage reductions.

- **Weight Changes:** Significant weight loss can affect drug distribution and concentration. Dosage adjustments may be needed to ensure the medication is still effective and safe.

- **Symptom Management:** As symptoms change, medication dosages may need to be adjusted to provide optimal relief. For example, increasing pain may require a higher dose of pain medication.

- **Individual Response:** Each individual responds differently to medications. Dosage adjustments may be needed based on the individual's response and tolerance.

Changing Routes of Administration

- **Difficulty Swallowing:** As swallowing becomes more difficult, alternative routes of administration may be necessary.

- **Nausea and Vomiting:** Oral medications may be poorly tolerated if the individual is experiencing nausea or vomiting.

- **Changes in Consciousness:** If the individual's level of consciousness declines, they may no longer be able to safely take oral medications.

- **Available Routes:** Common alternative routes include:

- **Rectal:** Some medications can be administered rectally via suppositories.

- **Transdermal:** Medications can be absorbed through the skin using patches.

- **Sublingual:** Medications can be placed under the tongue to dissolve.

- **Subcutaneous or Intravenous:** These routes require injections and are usually administered by a healthcare professional, but in some cases, family members may be trained.

- **Consult with the Healthcare Team:** It's crucial to consult with the healthcare team before changing the route of administration. They can determine the most appropriate route and provide instructions on how to administer the medication safely.

Managing Side Effects

- **Common Side Effects:** Be aware of the potential side effects of each medication. Common side effects in end-of-life care include nausea, vomiting, constipation, drowsiness, confusion, and dry mouth.

- **Proactive Management:** Anticipate and proactively manage potential side effects. For example, if constipation is a common side effect of a medication, implement preventative measures such as increasing fluid intake (if appropriate) and using stool softeners as prescribed.

- **Symptom-Specific Interventions:** If side effects occur, implement appropriate interventions. For nausea, antiemetics may be prescribed. For dry mouth, saliva substitutes or frequent sips of water may be helpful.

- **Reporting Side Effects:** Report any suspected side effects to the healthcare team promptly. They can assess the situation and make recommendations for managing the side effects or adjusting the medication regimen.

- **Non-Pharmacological Approaches:** Consider non-pharmacological approaches to managing side effects. For example, ginger can be helpful for nausea, and relaxation techniques can help with anxiety.

Important Considerations for Medication Administration

- **Focus on Comfort:** The primary goal of medication administration at the end of life is to manage symptoms and ensure comfort.

- **Minimize Burden:** Choose the least invasive and most convenient route of administration whenever possible.

- **Simplify Regimens:** Simplify medication regimens as much as possible to reduce the burden on caregivers and the individual.

- **Regular Review:** Regularly review the medication list with the healthcare team to ensure that all medications are still appropriate and necessary.

- **Medication Reconciliation:** Ensure that all medications, including prescription medications, over-the-counter medications, and supplements, are documented and reviewed by the healthcare team.

- **Proper Storage:** Store medications safely and securely, following the manufacturer's instructions.

- **Disposal of Medications:** Dispose of unused or expired medications properly, following local guidelines.

- administration.

Proper Storage of Medications

Proper medication storage is important for maintaining medication effectiveness and safety, especially during end-of-life care when individuals may be more vulnerable to adverse effects. Here's a guide to proper medication storage:

General Guidelines:

- **Cool, Dry Place:** Most medications should be stored at room temperature, generally between

59°F and 77°F (15°C and 25°C), in a cool, dry place. Avoid storing medications in bathrooms or near sources of heat and moisture, as these conditions can degrade the medication.

- **Original Containers:** Keep medications in their original containers with the labels intact. This helps prevent mix-ups and ensures you have access to important information, such as the medication name, dosage, expiration date, and any specific storage instructions.

- **Out of Reach of Children and Pets:** Store all medications out of the reach and sight of children and pets. Consider using child-resistant containers or storing medications in a locked cabinet.

- **Away from Direct Sunlight:** Exposure to direct sunlight can damage some medications. Store medications in a dark or shaded area.

- **Check Expiration Dates:** Regularly check the expiration dates on all medications and discard any expired medications. Expired medications may be less effective or even harmful.

- **Follow Specific Instructions:** Some medications may have specific storage requirements, such as refrigeration. Always read the medication label and follow any specific storage instructions provided by the pharmacist or healthcare provider.

Specific Storage Considerations

- **Refrigerated Medications:** Medications that require refrigeration should be stored in the refrigerator, typically between 36°F and 46°F (2°C and 8°C). Do not freeze medications unless specifically instructed to do so.

- **Insulin:** Insulin should be stored in the refrigerator, but it can be kept at room temperature for up to 28 days once opened. Avoid exposing insulin to extreme temperatures or direct sunlight.

- **Liquid Medications:** Liquid medications may have specific storage requirements. Some may need to be refrigerated, while others should be stored at room temperature. Always check the label for instructions.

- **Medication in Multi-Dose Containers:** If you have a liquid medication in a multi-dose container, note the date it was opened and discard any remaining medication after the recommended time frame.

- **Medication in Blister Packs:** Keep medications in their original blister packs until you are ready to take them. This helps protect the medication from moisture and contamination.

Disposing of Medications

- **Follow Local Guidelines:** Follow local guidelines for disposing of unused or expired medications. Many communities have drug take-back programs or designated disposal sites.

- **Do Not Flush Down the Toilet:** Avoid flushing medications down the toilet unless specifically instructed to do so. This can contaminate the water supply.

- **Mix with Undesirable Substance:** If you cannot dispose of medications through a take-back program, mix them with an undesirable substance, such as coffee grounds or kitty litter, seal them in a plastic bag, and discard them in the trash.

Travel Considerations

- **Carry Medications with You:** When traveling, carry medications in your carry-on luggage to avoid exposure to extreme temperatures in the cargo hold.

- **Keep Medications in Original Containers:** Keep medications in their original containers with the labels intact.

- **Carry a Medication List:** Carry a list of all your medications, including the names, dosages, and prescribing healthcare providers.

Communication with the Healthcare Team

- **Ask Questions:** If you have any questions about medication storage, don't hesitate to ask your pharmacist or healthcare provider for clarification.

- **Inform of any Changes:** Inform your healthcare team of any changes in your medication storage practices or any concerns about medication effectiveness or safety.

By following these guidelines for proper medication storage, caregivers can help ensure the safety and effectiveness of medications.

Recognizing Possible Side Effects

As the body's systems slow down, individuals become more susceptible to adverse drug reactions, and it's essential to be vigilant and proactive in monitoring for any changes.

Why Recognizing Side Effects is Important

- **Improved Comfort:** Identifying and managing side effects can significantly improve the individual's comfort and quality of life.

- **Prevention of Complications:** Prompt recognition and intervention can prevent serious complications related to medication side effects.

- **Medication Adjustments:** Recognizing side effects allows for timely dosage adjustments or medication changes by the healthcare team.

- **Enhanced Communication:** Being aware of potential side effects enables caregivers to communicate effectively with the healthcare team, ensuring optimal medication management.

Common Side Effects

- **Gastrointestinal Issues**

    o **Nausea and Vomiting:** Many medications, especially opioids, can cause nausea and vomiting.

    o **Constipation:** Opioids and other medications can slow down the digestive system, leading to constipation.

    o **Diarrhea:** Some medications can cause diarrhea.

- **Neurological Effects**

    o **Drowsiness and Sedation:** Many medications can cause drowsiness, especially in older adults or when taken in combination with other medications.

    o **Confusion and Delirium:** Changes in cognition, including confusion, delirium, or hallucinations, can be side effects of certain medications.

- o **Dizziness and Lightheadedness:** Some medications can cause dizziness or lightheadedness, increasing the risk of falls.

- **Respiratory Issues**

  - o **Respiratory Depression:** Opioids can slow down breathing, and in some cases, lead to respiratory depression, especially at higher doses or in individuals with pre-existing respiratory conditions.

- **Other Common Side Effects**

  - o **Dry Mouth:** Many medications can cause dry mouth, which can be uncomfortable and contribute to oral health problems.

  - o **Loss of Appetite:** Some medications can decrease appetite or alter taste, leading to reduced food intake.

  - o **Skin Issues:** Rashes, itching, or other skin irritations can be side effects of certain medications.

  - o **Fatigue:** Many medications can contribute to fatigue or weakness.

How to Recognize Side Effects

- **Be Aware of Medications:** Know the names, dosages, purposes, and potential side effects of all medications being taken.

- **Observe Changes:** Pay close attention to any changes in the individual's physical or mental state, including new symptoms or changes in existing symptoms.

- **Ask Questions:** If you are unsure whether a symptom is related to a medication, don't hesitate to ask the healthcare team.

- **Keep a Medication Log:** Keep a record of all medications being taken, including the dosage, frequency, and any observed side effects.

- **Consider Drug Interactions:** Be aware that taking multiple medications can increase the risk of side effects and drug interactions.

What to Do if You Suspect a Side Effect

- **Report to the Healthcare Team:** Contact the healthcare team promptly if you suspect a medication side effect. Provide them with detailed information about the observed symptoms, including when they started and how severe they are.

- **Do Not Stop Medication Abruptly:** Do not stop or change the dosage of any medication without consulting with the healthcare team.

- **Follow Instructions:** Follow the healthcare team's instructions for managing the side effect. This may involve adjusting the dosage, changing the medication, or using other interventions to alleviate the symptoms.

Communication with the Healthcare Team

- **Open Communication:** Maintain open and ongoing communication with the healthcare team about any concerns regarding medication side effects.

- **Accurate Information:** Provide accurate and detailed information about the observed symptoms.

- **Collaboration:** Work collaboratively with the healthcare team to ensure safe and effective medication management.

Important Considerations

- **Individual Variability:** Each individual responds differently to medications. Some people may experience side effects that are not listed or are less common.

- **Multiple Medications:** Individuals at the end of life often take multiple medications, increasing the risk of side effects and drug interactions.

- **Changes in Condition:** As the individual's condition changes, their response to medications may also change, requiring adjustments in dosage or medication.

Medication administration can be challenging, but by working closely with the healthcare team, being aware of potential complications, and prioritizing comfort, caregivers can ensure their loved ones receive safe and effective medication management.

Part 3
Emotional and Spiritual Support

Chapter 10

Emotional Support for the Dying Loved One

Providing emotional comfort is one of the most profound and meaningful aspects of caregiving. It involves offering presence, support, and understanding during a time of significant transition and vulnerability. It's about creating a space where the individual feels safe, loved, and heard.

Key Elements of Emotional Comfort

- **Presence:** Simply being present with the individual can be incredibly comforting. Your physical presence conveys love, support, and companionship. It's not always about doing something, but simply being there.

- **Active Listening:** Listen attentively to their concerns, fears, and hopes. Avoid interrupting or offering unsolicited advice. Focus on truly hearing what they are saying, both verbally and nonverbally.

- **Empathy and Understanding:** Try to understand the individual's emotional experience. Acknowledge their feelings without judgment. Let them know that their feelings are valid and that you are there for them.

- **Reassurance:** Offer reassurance and comfort. Let them know that they are not alone and that you will be there for them throughout this journey.

- **Respect and Dignity:** Treat the individual with respect and dignity throughout the end-of-life process. Honor their wishes and preferences as much as possible.

- **Honest and Open Communication:** Encourage open and honest communication. Create a safe space where they can express their fears, concerns, and hopes without feeling judged.

- **Emotional Support:** Provide emotional support without trying to "fix" their emotions. Allow them to express their feelings, whether they are sadness, anger, fear, or acceptance.

- **Meaningful Connections:** Facilitate meaningful connections with family and friends. Help them connect with loved ones in whatever way is most comfortable for them, whether it's through visits, phone calls, letters, or video chats.

- **Reminiscence:** Sharing memories and stories can be a comforting and meaningful way to connect with the individual. Looking through photos or listening to music from their past can evoke positive emotions and provide a sense of connection to their life.

- **Spiritual Support:** If the individual is religious or spiritual, provide access to spiritual resources, such as clergy, spiritual advisors, or sacred texts. Support their spiritual practices and beliefs.

- **Hope and Meaning:** Even at the end of life, there can be a sense of hope and meaning. Help the individual find meaning in their life and legacy. Focus on the positive aspects of their life and the impact they have had on others.

- **Comforting Touch:** Gentle touch, such as holding hands or stroking their arm, can be incredibly comforting and reassuring.

- **Creating a Peaceful Atmosphere:** A calm and peaceful environment can help reduce anxiety and promote relaxation. This might involve playing soft music, dimming the lights, or simply spending quiet time together.

Addressing Specific Emotional Needs

Fear of Dying

Acknowledge and validate their fear. Offer reassurance and explore their concerns. Focus on the present moment and what can be done to ensure comfort and peace.

Supporting someone through their fear of dying is a delicate and deeply important aspect of caregiving. It requires empathy, patience, and a willingness to explore difficult emotions.

Understanding the Fear

- **Acknowledge and Validate:** Recognize that fear of dying is a natural and valid emotion. Don't dismiss or minimize their fears. Let them know it's okay to feel scared.

- **Explore the Source:** Gently try to understand the root of their fear. Are they afraid of the unknown, the process of dying, leaving loved ones behind, pain, or something else? Understanding the specific fear can help you tailor your support.

- **Common Fears:** Some common fears associated with death include:

    - **Fear of the unknown:** What happens after death?
    - **Fear of the dying process:** Will it be painful? Will I be alone?
    - **Fear of separation from loved ones:** What will happen to my family?
    - **Fear of losing control:** Over their body, their mind, their life.
    - **Fear of non-existence:** The idea of ceasing to exist can be frightening.

Providing Emotional Support

- **Presence:** Simply being present with the individual can be incredibly comforting. Your calm and supportive presence conveys love and reassurance.

- **Active Listening:** Listen attentively and empathetically to their fears. Let them express their feelings without interruption or judgment. Focus on truly hearing what they are saying, both verbally and nonverbally.

- **Open and Honest Communication:** Create a safe space for open and honest conversations about death and dying. Encourage them to express their fears and concerns without feeling ashamed or embarrassed.

- **Empathy and Compassion:** Show empathy and compassion for their fears. Acknowledge their feelings and let them know you understand their struggle.

- **Reassurance:** Offer reassurance and comfort. Let them know they are not alone and that you will be there for them.

- **Avoid Clichés:** Avoid offering empty clichés or platitudes, such as "Everything will be okay" or "You'll be in a better place." These can minimize their fears and make them feel unheard.

- **Focus on the Present:** Gently guide their attention to the present moment. Focus on what is happening now and what can be done to ensure comfort and peace in the present.

- **Meaning and Purpose:** Help them find meaning and purpose in their life, even as death approaches. Reminiscing about positive memories and accomplishments can be helpful.

- **Hope and Possibility:** While acknowledging the reality of death, it's also important to offer hope. Hope for comfort, hope for connection, hope for a peaceful transition.

- **Spiritual Support:** If the individual is religious or spiritual, support their beliefs and practices. Offer access to spiritual resources, such as clergy, spiritual advisors, or sacred texts.

- **Professional Help:** If the fear is overwhelming or causing significant distress, encourage them to seek professional help from a therapist, counselor, or chaplain.

Things to Say (and How to Say Them)

- "I'm here with you. I'm listening." (Simple presence is often the most powerful support.)

- "It's understandable to feel scared. This is a difficult time." (Validating their feelings.)

- "What are you most afraid of?" (Encouraging them to express their specific fears.)

- "I'm here to support you in any way I can." (Offering practical and emotional support.)

- "Tell me about your concerns." (Creating a safe space for open communication.)

- "I'm not sure what happens after death, but I'm here with you now." (Honesty and acknowledging the unknown.)

- "Let's focus on making you as comfortable as possible." (Shifting the focus to present comfort.)

- "What brings you comfort right now?" (Focusing on their immediate needs and preferences.)

Important Considerations

- **Individual Differences:** Each person's experience with fear of dying is unique. Be sensitive to their individual needs and preferences.

- **Nonverbal Communication:** Pay attention to nonverbal cues, such as facial expressions and body language. Offer comfort through gentle touch, eye contact, and a calm demeanor.

- **Self-Care for Caregivers:** Supporting someone through their fear of dying can be emotionally challenging. Remember to prioritize your own well-being and seek support when needed.

Supporting someone through their fear of dying is a sacred and profound responsibility. By offering presence, empathy, and understanding, you can help them navigate this difficult time with greater peace and acceptance.

Grief and Loss

Allow the individual to express their grief and loss. Acknowledge their pain and offer support.

Understanding Grief and Loss at End of Life

- **Anticipatory Grief:** The person may be grieving losses they are experiencing *before* death, such as loss of physical abilities, independence, roles, relationships, and the life they knew.

- **Multiple Losses:** They may be grieving past losses resurfacing, losses related to their illness, and the ultimate loss of their own life.

- **Unique Experience:** Grief is a highly individual process. There is no right or wrong way to grieve, and everyone experiences loss differently.

- **Fluctuating Emotions:** Expect a wide range of emotions, including sadness, anger, fear, denial, acceptance, and everything in between. These emotions may come in waves and change rapidly.

How to Help

- **Presence:** Simply being present with the individual can be incredibly comforting. Your calm and supportive presence conveys love and reassurance.

- **Active Listening:** Listen attentively and empathetically to their feelings. Avoid interrupting or offering unsolicited advice. Focus on truly hearing what they are saying, both verbally and nonverbally.

- **Acknowledge and Validate:** Acknowledge their pain and let them know their feelings are valid. Avoid minimizing their grief or trying to "fix" it.

- **Create a Safe Space:** Offer a calm, supportive, and non-judgmental environment where they feel comfortable expressing their emotions without fear of criticism or dismissal.

- **Encourage Expression:** Encourage them to express their grief in whatever way feels natural to them, whether it's through talking, crying, writing, art, music, or spending time in nature.

- **Be Patient:** Grief takes time. Be patient and allow them to grieve at their own pace. Don't pressure them to "move on" or "get over it."

- **Offer Practical Support:** Offer practical assistance with daily tasks, errands, or other needs. This can alleviate some stress and allow them to focus on their emotional needs.

- **Respect Silence:** Sometimes, the most supportive thing you can do is simply be present in silence. Allow them space to process their emotions without pressure to talk.

- **Physical Comfort:** Gentle touch, such as holding hands or stroking their arm, can be incredibly comforting.

- **Spiritual Support:** If the individual is religious or spiritual, support their beliefs and practices. Offer access to spiritual resources, such as clergy, spiritual advisors, or sacred texts.

- **Memory Sharing:** Reminiscing about positive memories and sharing stories can be a way to honor their life and acknowledge their legacy.

- **Professional Support:** If their grief is overwhelming or causing significant distress, encourage them to seek professional help from a therapist, counselor, or chaplain.

Things to Say (and How to Say Them)

- "I'm so sorry you're going through this." (Simple and heartfelt.)

- "It's okay to feel sad/angry/scared/etc." (Validating their emotions.)

- "I'm here for you. I'm listening." (Offering presence and support.)

- "Tell me how you're feeling." (Encouraging open communication.)

- "I can only imagine how difficult this must be." (Acknowledging their pain.)

- "There's no right or wrong way to grieve." (Normalizing their experience.)

- "It's okay to cry." (Allowing for emotional expression.)

- "I'm here to listen whenever you're ready to talk." (Offering ongoing support.)

Things to Avoid Saying

- "You'll get over it." (Minimizes their pain and implies a timeline for grief.)

- "It's for the best." (May feel dismissive of their loss.)

- "You need to be strong." (Puts pressure on them to suppress emotions.)

- "I know how you feel." (Unless you've experienced a very similar loss, this can feel dismissive.)

- "At least they're not suffering anymore." (While well-intentioned, it may not be comforting to everyone.)

Important Considerations

- **Individual Differences:** Everyone grieves differently. Be sensitive to their unique needs and preferences.

Anger

If the individual is experiencing anger, allow them to express it without judgment. Try to understand the underlying reasons for their anger and offer compassion.

Anger during end-of-life care is a natural, albeit challenging, emotion. It can stem from a variety of sources, including the unfairness of the situation, loss of control, pain, fear, or unresolved issues. Helping someone navigate this anger requires patience, empathy, and a safe space for them to express their feelings without judgment.

Understanding the Anger

- **Acknowledge and Validate:** Recognize that anger is a normal response to loss, suffering, and the end of life. Don't dismiss or minimize their anger. Let them know it's okay to feel angry.

- **Explore the Source:** Gently try to understand the root of their anger. Is it directed at the illness, the healthcare system, family members, themselves, or something else entirely? Understanding the target of their anger can help you tailor your support.

- **Underlying Emotions:** Anger often masks other emotions, such as fear, sadness, or grief. Explore what might be underlying the anger.

- **Loss of Control:** Terminal illness often involves a loss of control over one's body, life, and future. Anger can be a way of expressing this frustration.

- **Unfairness:** The individual may feel that their situation is unfair, leading to resentment and anger.

How to Help

- **Presence:** Simply being present with the individual can be incredibly comforting. Your calm and supportive presence conveys love and reassurance.

- **Active Listening:** Listen attentively and empathetically to their anger. Let them express their feelings without interruption or judgment. Focus on truly hearing what they are saying, both verbally and nonverbally.

- **Create a Safe Space:** Offer a calm, supportive, and non-judgmental environment where they feel comfortable expressing their anger without fear of criticism or retaliation.

- **Empathy and Compassion:** Show empathy and compassion for their anger. Acknowledge their pain and frustration.

- **Avoid Taking it Personally:** Remember that their anger is likely not directed at you personally, even if it feels that way. Try not to take it personally and focus on providing support.

- **Don't Try to Fix It:** You can't "fix" their anger, but you can offer support and understanding. Don't try to argue with them or tell them how they should feel.

- **Respect Their Need for Space:** Sometimes, the most helpful thing you can do is give them space to process their anger. Let them know you're there for them when they're ready to talk.

- **Help Them Find Healthy Outlets:** Encourage them to find healthy ways to express their anger, such as talking to a therapist, writing in a journal, or engaging in creative activities.

- **Focus on Comfort:** Shift the focus to ensuring their physical comfort and managing any pain or other symptoms that may be contributing to their anger.

- **Spiritual Support:** If the individual is religious or spiritual, connect them with a chaplain, spiritual advisor, or other spiritual resources.

- **Professional Support:** If the anger is overwhelming or causing significant distress, encourage them to seek professional help from a therapist or counselor.

Things to Say (and How to Say Them)

- "I can see that you're feeling angry." (Acknowledging their emotion.)

- "It's understandable to feel angry in this situation." (Validating their feeling.)

- "I'm here for you. I'm listening." (Offering presence and support.)

- "Tell me what's making you feel so angry." (Encouraging them to express their feelings.)

- "It's okay to feel angry. You don't have to hold it in." (Normalizing their anger.)

- "I'm not going to try to change how you feel, but I'm here to listen if you want to talk." (Offering support without judgment.)

Things to Avoid Saying:

- "You shouldn't feel that way." (Invalidating their emotions.)

- "Calm down." (Often has the opposite effect.)

- "It could be worse." (Minimizing their pain.)

- "Just try to be positive." (Dismissive of their feelings.)

Important Considerations

- **Safety:** If the individual's anger becomes verbally abusive or threatening, it's important to set boundaries and prioritize your own safety. Seek help from other caregivers or healthcare professionals if necessary.

Depression

Depression is common at the end of life. Talk to the healthcare team about treatment options, which may include medication or counseling.

Recognizing Depression at End of Life

It's important to differentiate between sadness, which is a natural response to loss and the dying process, and clinical depression, which is a medical condition. Some common signs of depression include:

- **Persistent Sadness:** A prolonged period of low mood that doesn't lift.

- **Loss of Interest:** Diminished interest in activities they once enjoyed.

- **Changes in Sleep:** Difficulty sleeping or sleeping excessively.

- **Changes in Appetite:** Significant changes in eating habits, either eating much more or much less than usual.

- **Fatigue:** Persistent tiredness and lack of energy.

- **Feelings of Worthlessness or Guilt:** Expressing feelings of worthlessness, hopelessness, or excessive guilt.

- **Social Withdrawal:** Withdrawing from social interactions and isolating themselves.

- **Irritability or Agitation:** Increased irritability, restlessness, or agitation.

- **Difficulty Concentrating:** Problems with focus, memory, or decision-making.

- **Thoughts of Death or Suicide:** Expressing thoughts about death or suicide.

How to Help

- **Acknowledge and Validate:** Acknowledge their feelings and let them know it's okay to feel depressed. Avoid minimizing their emotions or telling them to "snap out of it."

- **Active Listening:** Listen attentively and empathetically to what they have to say. Create a safe space for them to express their feelings without judgment.

- **Empathy and Compassion:** Show empathy and compassion for their suffering. Let them know you understand they are going through a difficult time.

- **Encourage Communication:** Encourage them to talk about their feelings with you, other loved ones, or a healthcare professional.

- **Offer Support:** Offer practical support, such as helping with daily tasks, running errands, or providing transportation to medical appointments.

- **Promote Comfort:** Create a comfortable and peaceful environment. Offer gentle touch, play soothing music, or engage in other activities that bring them comfort.

- **Social Connection:** Encourage social interaction, even if it's just spending time with a loved one or engaging in a favorite hobby.

- **Spiritual Support:** If the individual is religious or spiritual, connect them with a chaplain, spiritual advisor, or other spiritual resources.

- **Professional Help:** Encourage them to seek professional help from a therapist, counselor, or psychiatrist. Depression is a treatable condition, even at the end of life.

Important Considerations

- **Underlying Medical Conditions:** Be aware that some medical conditions or medications can contribute to depression. Discuss any concerns with the healthcare team.

- **Grief vs. Depression:** It can be challenging to distinguish between normal grief and clinical depression. If you are unsure, consult with a healthcare professional.

- **Suicidal Ideation:** If the individual expresses thoughts of death or suicide, it's crucial to take it seriously and seek immediate professional help.

- **Self-Care for Caregivers:** Supporting someone with depression can be emotionally draining. Remember to prioritize your own well-being and seek support when needed.

Working with the Healthcare Team

- **Communicate Concerns:** Share your observations and concerns with the healthcare team. They can assess the individual's symptoms and recommend appropriate interventions.

- **Medication Management:** Discuss medication options with the healthcare team. Antidepressants can be effective in treating depression, even at the end of life.

- **Therapy and Counseling:** Explore therapy or counseling options. A therapist can provide emotional support and help the individual cope with their depression.

Remember

- **Depression is a medical condition:** It's not a sign of weakness or a character flaw.

- **Help is available:** There are effective treatments for depression, even at the end of life.

- **You are not alone:** Many resources are available to support individuals and families dealing with depression during end-of-life care.

Chapter 11

Spiritual Care

Spiritual support is a instrumental aspect of holistic care. It addresses the individual's fundamental needs for meaning, purpose, connection, and transcendence as they face the end of their life journey. It acknowledges that human beings are not just physical and emotional beings, but also spiritual beings with unique needs and beliefs.

Why Spiritual Support Matters

- **Meaning and Purpose:** End-of-life care often prompts deep reflection on the meaning of life and the individual's legacy. Spiritual support can help them explore these questions, find meaning in their experiences, and achieve a sense of purpose, even in the face of death.

- **Hope and Transcendence:** Spiritual beliefs can provide hope and a sense of transcendence, offering comfort and solace in the face of the unknown. It can help individuals find peace and acceptance as they approach death.

- **Connection and Belonging:** Spiritual communities and practices can provide a sense of connection and belonging, which can be especially important during a time of isolation or vulnerability. It can also connect them to something larger than themselves.

- **Forgiveness and Reconciliation:** Spiritual support can help individuals address issues of forgiveness, both of themselves and others. It can facilitate reconciliation and bring peace to unresolved relationships.

- **Comfort and Peace:** Spiritual practices, such as prayer, meditation, or rituals, can provide comfort and a sense of peace during a time of great stress and uncertainty.

- **Grief and Loss:** Spiritual beliefs can offer a framework for understanding death and loss, helping individuals and their families navigate the grieving process.

- **Respecting Individual Beliefs:** Spiritual support is not about imposing religious views. It's about respecting the individual's own beliefs, values, and practices, whether they are religious, agnostic, or atheist.

How to Provide Spiritual Support

- **Active Listening:** Listen attentively and empathetically to the individual's spiritual concerns. Create a safe space for them to express their beliefs, fears, and hopes.

- **Explore Their Beliefs:** Ask open-ended questions about their spiritual beliefs and practices. What gives their life meaning? What do they believe about death and the afterlife?

- **Facilitate Connections:** Connect the individual with spiritual resources that are meaningful to them, such as clergy, spiritual advisors, or members of their faith community.

- **Support Spiritual Practices:** Support their spiritual practices, whether it's prayer, meditation, reading sacred texts, listening to religious music, or spending time in nature.

- **Respectful Presence:** Simply being present with the individual can be a profound form of spiritual support. Your calm and supportive presence conveys love, care, and companionship.

- **Create a Sacred Space:** Help them create a peaceful and sacred space where they can engage in their spiritual practices. This might involve setting up an altar, playing calming music, or displaying meaningful objects.

- **Offer Rituals and Sacraments:** If appropriate, offer to assist with religious rituals or sacraments, such as communion, anointing of the sick, or last rites.

- **Address Spiritual Distress:** Be aware of signs of spiritual distress, such as feelings of abandonment, meaninglessness, or guilt. Offer support and connect them with appropriate resources.

- **Collaboration with Chaplaincy/Spiritual Care:** If the individual is in a hospital or care facility, collaborate with the chaplaincy or spiritual care department. They are trained to provide spiritual support to individuals of all faiths and backgrounds.

Important Considerations

- **Respect Individual Differences:** Be sensitive to the individual's unique spiritual needs and preferences. Avoid making assumptions about their beliefs or imposing your own views.

- **Cultural Sensitivity:** Be mindful of cultural differences in spiritual beliefs and practices.

- **No Proselytizing:** Do not attempt to convert the individual to your own religious beliefs.

- **Focus on the Individual:** The goal is to support the individual's spiritual journey, not to promote any particular religion or belief system.

Activities that Provide Spiritual Support

For those who are religious

- **Prayer:** Offer to pray with them, or if they prefer, read prayers aloud.

- **Religious Texts:** Read passages from their holy book or other inspirational writings.

- **Music:** Play hymns or religious music that are significant to them.

- **Rituals:** Assist with religious rituals or sacraments they may wish to receive, such as communion, anointing of the sick, or last rites.

- **Visits from Clergy:** Facilitate visits from their pastor, priest, rabbi, imam, or other religious leader.

For those who are spiritual but not religious

- **Nature:** Spend time in nature, if possible. The beauty and tranquility of the natural world can be very comforting.

- **Meditation:** Guide them through a meditation or mindfulness exercise.

- **Gratitude Practice:** Help them reflect on the positive aspects of their life and express gratitude for the good things they have experienced.

- **Legacy Projects:** Help them create a legacy project, such as a memory book, a video recording, or a piece of art. This can be a way to leave a lasting impact on their loved ones.

- **Meaningful Conversations:** Engage in deep conversations about life, death, and what matters most to them.

- **Music:** Play music that is calming, uplifting, or has special meaning to them.

- **Art:** Engage in art activities, such as painting, drawing, or sculpting.

- **Journaling:** Encourage them to write down their thoughts and feelings in a journal.

For those who are agnostic or atheist

- **Meaning-Making Activities:** Help them explore what gives their life meaning and purpose. This could involve reflecting on their relationships, accomplishments, or contributions to the world.

- **Connection with Loved Ones:** Facilitate meaningful connections with family and friends. Spending time with loved ones can be a source of great comfort and joy.

- **Reminiscence:** Share memories and stories about their life. Looking through photos or listening to music from their past can be a powerful way to connect with their life and legacy.

- **Nature:** Spending time in nature can be a source of peace and inspiration for anyone, regardless of their beliefs.

- **Acts of Kindness:** Engaging in acts of kindness or helping others can bring a sense of purpose and fulfillment.

- **Music and Art:** Music and art can be powerful ways to express emotions and connect with something larger than oneself.

General Activities that can be Supportive

- **Reading:** Reading inspirational or thought-provoking books or poems.

- **Listening to Music:** Music can be incredibly soothing and can evoke powerful emotions and memories.

- **Spending Time with Loved Ones:** Connecting with family and friends can provide a sense of love, belonging, and support.

- **Quiet Reflection:** Spending time in quiet reflection or meditation can help them process their thoughts and feelings.

- **Expressing Gratitude:** Focusing on the positive aspects of their life and expressing gratitude can bring a sense of peace and contentment.

Important Considerations

- **Respect Individual Preferences:** Always respect the individual's unique spiritual beliefs and practices. Avoid imposing your own views or making assumptions about their beliefs.

- **Offer, Don't Impose:** Offer spiritual support, but don't force it. Let the individual guide the process and choose what activities are most meaningful to them.

- **Be Present:** Sometimes, the most important thing you can do is simply be present with the person, offering your love and support.

Remember, spiritual support is about honoring the individual's unique journey and helping them find comfort, meaning, and connection during this time.

Chapter 12

Addressing Unfinished Business

People can have a wide range of "unfinished business" at the end of life. It's often a complex mix of emotional, relational, practical, and spiritual matters. Here are some common categories and examples:

Relational Issues

- **Broken or Strained Relationships:** This could involve family members, friends, or even past romantic partners. The unfinished business might be a need to apologize, forgive, seek forgiveness, or simply reconnect.

- **Unexpressed Love or Gratitude:** People may regret not expressing their love and appreciation to important people in their lives.

- **Unresolved Conflicts:** Lingering disagreements, arguments, or misunderstandings can weigh heavily on someone's mind.

- **Saying Goodbye:** Not having the chance to say goodbye properly to loved ones who have already passed.

Emotional Issues

- **Regrets:** Regrets about past choices, missed opportunities, or things left undone. This could be related to career, relationships, travel, or personal growth.

- **Guilt:** Guilt over past actions, mistakes, or perceived failures.

- **Unforgiveness:** Holding onto resentment, anger, or bitterness towards others or even oneself.

- **Fear:** Fear of the unknown, the dying process, pain, or leaving loved ones behind.

- **Unexpressed Emotions:** Not having adequately expressed sadness, joy, anger, or other important emotions.

Practical Matters

- **Financial Affairs:** Unresolved financial matters, such as unpaid bills, an unclear will, or concerns about the financial security of loved ones.

- **Legal Issues:** Unfinished legal matters, such as property ownership, custody arrangements, or pending lawsuits.

- **Personal Belongings:** Concerns about what will happen to cherished possessions or how they will be distributed.

- **Funeral Arrangements:** Not having made funeral or memorial service arrangements.

Spiritual Concerns

- **Meaning and Purpose:** Questioning the meaning and purpose of life, especially in the face of death.

- **Spiritual Reconciliation:** Seeking reconciliation with a higher power or finding peace with one's spiritual beliefs.

- **Fear of Death or the Afterlife:** Anxiety or fear about what happens after death.

- **Unresolved Spiritual Questions:** Lingering questions about faith, the nature of existence, or the meaning of suffering.

Personal Goals and Dreams

- **Unfulfilled Ambitions:** Regrets about not achieving certain goals or dreams, whether related to career, education, travel, or personal growth.

- **Unfinished Projects:** Desire to complete unfinished projects, such as writing a book, painting a picture, or building something.

- **Missed Opportunities:** Regrets about not taking certain chances or pursuing passions.

It's important to remember that everyone's "unfinished business" is unique to them. What one person considers important, another might not. The key is to offer a supportive and non-judgmental space for individuals to explore these issues and address them to the best of their ability.

Addressing unfinished business is incredibly important for a person's emotional and spiritual well-being. Here's why:

- **Peace of Mind:** Resolving lingering issues, whether with relationships, regrets, or unfulfilled goals, can bring a sense of peace and closure. It allows the individual to let go of burdens and focus on the present moment.

- **Reduced Anxiety:** Unfinished business can create anxiety and fear about the unknown. By addressing these issues, individuals can reduce their anxiety and feel more at peace with the dying process.

- **Improved Emotional Well-being:** Resolving conflicts, expressing love and forgiveness, and completing important tasks can lead to improved emotional well-being. It can reduce feelings of guilt, regret, and resentment.

- **Enhanced Spiritual Well-being:** Addressing spiritual concerns, such as seeking forgiveness or reconciliation, can bring a sense of spiritual peace and connection. It can help individuals find meaning and purpose in their lives, even as they face death.

- **Increased Sense of Control:** At a time when many things feel out of control, addressing unfinished business can give individuals a sense of agency and control over their lives. It allows them to actively participate in their end-of-life care.

- **Strengthened Relationships:** Addressing unfinished business with loved ones can strengthen relationships and create lasting memories. It can be a way to express love, gratitude, and appreciation.

- **Legacy and Remembrance:** Completing important tasks or creating a legacy project can provide a sense of purpose and leave a lasting impact on loved ones. It can be a way to ensure their life and values are remembered.

Ultimately, addressing unfinished business is about helping individuals find peace, comfort, and closure as they approach the end of their lives. It's a way to honor their life journey and support them in making the most of their remaining time.

Forgiveness

Forgiveness, both given and received, holds immense

importance at the end of life for several profound reasons:

- **Emotional and Spiritual Peace:** Holding onto resentment, anger, or bitterness can create emotional and spiritual turmoil. Forgiveness offers a pathway to release these negative emotions, allowing for a sense of peace and tranquility as death approaches. It clears the heart and mind, creating space for more positive emotions like love, gratitude, and acceptance.

- **Reduced Burden:** Carrying the weight of unresolved conflict or unforgiven actions can be a heavy burden. Forgiveness lightens this load, freeing the individual from emotional baggage that can hinder their ability to experience peace and comfort in their final days.

- **Improved Relationships:** Forgiveness can mend broken relationships or heal strained ones. It opens the door for reconciliation, reconciliation can bring immense comfort and a sense of closure, not only for the dying person but also for their loved ones. It can mend rifts and create a sense of unity in the family.

- **Self-Forgiveness:** Often, the hardest person to forgive is oneself. Self-forgiveness is crucial for releasing guilt and regret. It allows individuals to accept their imperfections and find peace with their past actions. This is essential for self-acceptance and a sense of wholeness.

- **Focus on the Present:** Unresolved issues and lingering resentments can distract from the present moment, stealing precious time and energy from what truly matters at the end of life. Forgiveness helps shift the focus to the present, allowing individuals to cherish their remaining time and connect with loved ones.

- **Preparation for Transition:** Many believe that forgiveness is essential for a peaceful transition at the time of death. It allows individuals to let go of earthly burdens and approach death with a clear conscience and a sense of spiritual readiness.

- **Legacy of Love:** Choosing forgiveness sets a powerful example for loved ones. It leaves a legacy of love, compassion, and understanding, teaching future generations the importance of letting go of anger and embracing forgiveness.

- **Holistic Well-being:** Forgiveness is not just a spiritual act; it has a profound impact on emotional, psychological, and even physical well-being. Releasing anger and resentment can reduce stress, improve sleep, and promote overall health and comfort.

In essence, forgiveness at the end of life is about clearing the path for a more peaceful, meaningful, and loving transition. It's about letting go of the past, embracing the present, and preparing for whatever lies ahead with a heart at peace.

Reconciliation

Reconciliation holds significant importance for several interconnected reasons, contributing to emotional, spiritual, and relational well-being during a vulnerable time:

- **Emotional and Spiritual Peace:** Unresolved conflicts, hurt feelings, or broken relationships can create emotional and spiritual turmoil. Reconciliation offers a path to healing these wounds, bringing a sense of peace and closure. It releases the burden of anger, resentment, and regret, allowing for a more tranquil and accepting end-of-life experience.

- **Reduced Anxiety and Fear:** Unresolved issues can fuel anxiety and fear about death, particularly if they involve strained relationships or regrets. Reconciliation can alleviate these anxieties by mending rifts and creating a sense of connection and forgiveness. This can bring a sense of calm and preparedness.

- **Improved Relationships:** Reconciliation strengthens bonds with loved ones, creating a supportive and loving environment during the final stages of life. It allows for the expression of love, gratitude, and appreciation, fostering deeper connections and lasting memories. This is a gift not only for the dying person but also for those left behind.

- **Sense of Completion:** Reconciliation can provide a sense of completion, allowing individuals to feel they have addressed important matters before they die. This can be particularly important for those who value closure and want to leave their affairs in order, both practically and emotionally.

- **Focus on the Present Moment:** Unresolved conflicts can be a significant distraction, diverting energy and attention from the present moment. Reconciliation helps shift the focus to what truly matters: cherishing time with loved ones, expressing love, and finding peace in the present.

- **Preparation for Transition:** Many people find comfort in reconciling with loved ones as they prepare for the end of life. It can be a way of making peace with the past and preparing for whatever lies ahead, whether it's viewed from a spiritual or secular perspective.

- **Legacy of Love and Forgiveness:** Choosing reconciliation sets a powerful example for family and friends. It leaves a legacy of love, forgiveness, and the importance of mending relationships. This can be a valuable lesson for those grieving the loss.

- **Holistic Well-being:** Reconciliation has a positive impact on overall well-being, encompassing emotional, psychological, and even physical aspects. Releasing resentment and making amends can reduce stress, improve sleep, and promote a sense of overall comfort and peace.

Ways to Facilitate Reconciliation

Create a Safe and Supportive Environment

- **Privacy:** Ensure a private and comfortable setting where individuals can express themselves freely without fear of judgment or interruption.

- **Calm Atmosphere:** Create a calm and peaceful atmosphere. Minimize distractions and ensure a quiet space for conversation.

- **Emotional Support:** Offer emotional support and reassurance. Let individuals know that you are there for them and that their feelings are valid.

Encourage Open Communication

- **Open-Ended Questions:** Ask open-ended questions to encourage individuals to share their thoughts and feelings. Examples include:

  - "What is on your mind regarding your relationship with…?"

  - "What feelings do you have about this situation?"

  - "Is there anything you wish you had said or done differently?"

- **Active Listening:** Listen attentively and empathetically. Focus on truly understanding their perspective, even if you don't agree with it. Avoid interrupting or offering unsolicited advice.

- **Non-Judgmental Approach:** Approach the situation with a non-judgmental attitude. Avoid taking sides or placing blame. The goal is to facilitate healing, not to assign fault.

- **Validation of Feelings:** Validate their feelings, even if they are negative. Let them know it's okay to feel angry, hurt, or regretful.

Facilitate Communication Between Parties (If Desired)

- **Mediation:** If both parties are willing, you can act as a mediator to facilitate communication. Help them express their feelings and needs in a respectful way.

- **Letter Writing:** If direct communication is not possible or desired, encourage individuals to write letters expressing their feelings, offering forgiveness, or seeking forgiveness. You can offer to deliver the letters if needed.

- **Phone Calls or Video Chats:** Facilitate phone calls or video chats if both parties are comfortable with this form of communication.

- **Visits:** If possible and desired, arrange visits between individuals. This can be a powerful way to reconnect and reconcile.

Focus on Forgiveness

- **Explore the Meaning of Forgiveness:** Discuss the meaning of forgiveness and its potential benefits. Emphasize that forgiveness is not about condoning hurtful behavior, but about releasing resentment and finding peace.

- **Encourage Self-Forgiveness:** Help individuals explore self-forgiveness. Many people carry guilt and regret for past actions. Releasing this self-blame can be essential for reconciliation and peace.

- **Offer Forgiveness:** Encourage individuals to offer forgiveness to others, even if they have not received an apology. This can be a way to let go of anger and resentment.

Respect Boundaries and Wishes

- **Don't Force Reconciliation:** Never force anyone to reconcile if they are not willing or ready. Reconciliation is a personal choice and should not be pressured.

- **Respect Individual Preferences:** Respect individual preferences regarding how they want to communicate and with whom they want to reconcile.

- **Acknowledge Limitations:** Recognize that not all relationships can be fully reconciled. Sometimes, the most important thing is to offer forgiveness and let go.

Offer Spiritual Support (If Appropriate)

- **Connect with Spiritual Advisors:** If the individual is religious or spiritual, connect them with a chaplain, spiritual advisor, or other spiritual resources.

- **Support Spiritual Practices:** Support their spiritual practices, such as prayer, meditation, or rituals.

Self-Care for Caregivers

- **Emotional Support:** Supporting someone through reconciliation can be emotionally challenging. Remember to prioritize your own well-being and seek support if needed.

Important Considerations

- **Timing:** Be mindful of the timing. The individual's physical and emotional state may fluctuate. Choose a time when they are most comfortable and receptive.

- **Confidentiality:** Maintain confidentiality and respect the privacy of all parties involved.

- **Professional Help:** If the situation is complex or involves significant emotional distress, encourage individuals to seek professional help from a therapist or counselor.

In essence, reconciliation at the end of life is about healing relationships, finding peace with the past, and creating a loving and supportive environment for the individual and their loved ones. It's a gift of love, forgiveness, and connection that can bring comfort and meaning during a challenging time.

Love and Gratitude

Expressing love and gratitude at the end of life holds immense significance, both for the individual facing mortality and their loved ones. It's a profound way to address unfinished business and create lasting positive memories.

For the individual

- **Emotional Peace:** Expressing love and gratitude allows individuals to release any emotional burdens or regrets they may be carrying. It brings a sense of peace and closure, knowing they have shared their deepest feelings with those they cherish.

- **Sense of Completion:** Sharing love and appreciation can provide a sense of completion and fulfillment. It allows individuals to feel they have said what needs to be said, leaving no words unspoken.

- **Increased Well-being:** Expressing positive emotions like love and gratitude has been shown to have a positive impact on overall well-being. It can reduce stress, anxiety, and even pain.

- **Focus on the Positive:** Shifting the focus to love and gratitude can help individuals appreciate the good things in their lives, even as they face the end of their journey. It can bring joy and contentment during a challenging time.

For loved ones

- **Lasting Memories:** Expressions of love and gratitude create lasting memories that loved ones can cherish after the individual has passed away. These memories can be a source of comfort and strength during the grieving process.

- **Reassurance:** Hearing expressions of love and gratitude can provide reassurance and comfort to loved ones. It can help them know they are valued and appreciated.

- **Reduced Guilt and Regret:** Knowing that love and gratitude were shared can prevent future guilt and regret. It can provide peace of mind that important things were said and relationships were nurtured.

- **Strengthened Bonds:** Sharing love and gratitude can strengthen bonds between family and friends. It can create a deeper sense of connection and unity during a difficult time.

For both

- **Meaningful Connections:** Expressing love and gratitude fosters deeper and more meaningful connections between individuals and their loved ones. It creates a space for authentic communication and shared emotions.

- **A Legacy of Love:** These expressions leave a legacy of love and appreciation. They serve as a reminder of the importance of relationships and the power of positive emotions.

- **Preparation for Transition:** Sharing love and gratitude can be a way of preparing for the transition at the end of life. It allows both the individual and their loved ones to say goodbye with open hearts and a sense of peace.

In essence, expressing love and gratitude at the end of life is a precious gift. It's a way to honor relationships, create lasting memories, and find peace in the face of mortality. It allows individuals and their loved ones to connect on a deeper level and cherish the time they have together.

How you can facilitate this process

Create a Safe and Supportive Environment

- **Presence:** Simply being present with the individual, offering your calm and attentive presence, can be incredibly comforting. It conveys love and support without needing to say a word.

- **Active Listening:** Listen deeply and empathetically. Focus on truly understanding their perspective, even if you don't fully understand or agree with it. Avoid interrupting or offering unsolicited advice.

- **Non-Judgmental Space:** Create a safe and non-judgmental space where they feel comfortable expressing their feelings without fear of criticism or shame.

Encourage Reflection and Expression:

- **Open-Ended Questions:** Ask open-ended questions to prompt reflection and encourage them to share their thoughts and feelings. Examples include:

  - "Who are the most important people in your life, and why?"

  - "What are you most grateful for in your life?"

  - "What are some of your favorite memories with...?"

  - "Is there anything you want to say to...?"

- **Guided Reminiscence:** Help them reminisce about positive memories, significant relationships, and moments of joy. Looking through photos, listening to music, or revisiting special places (if possible) can be helpful.

- **Journaling:** Encourage them to write down their thoughts, feelings, and expressions of love and gratitude in a journal or letter.

- **Art and Creative Expression:** If writing isn't their preferred method, explore other creative outlets like painting, drawing, music, or even storytelling.

Facilitate Communication and Connection

- **Letter Writing:** Encourage them to write letters to loved ones expressing their love, gratitude, and appreciation. Offer to mail the letters if they are unable to do so themselves.

- **Phone Calls or Video Chats:** Facilitate phone calls or video chats with family and friends, especially those who may live far away.

- **Visits:** Arrange visits with loved ones whenever possible. These visits can be a powerful opportunity for connection, sharing, and expressing love and gratitude in person.

- **Sharing Stories:** Encourage them to share stories about their lives and relationships. This can be a way to express love and gratitude indirectly, by highlighting the positive impact others have had on their lives.

Focus on Love and Gratitude

- **Expressing Love:** Encourage them to express their love openly and freely to those they care about. Help them find the words if they are struggling.

- **Acknowledging Gratitude:** Help them identify and acknowledge the things they are grateful for in their lives. This can shift the focus from loss and sadness to appreciation and joy.

- **Thank You Notes:** Encourage them to write thank you notes to people who have made a difference in their lives.

Respect Boundaries and Wishes

- **No Pressure:** Never pressure anyone to express love or gratitude if they are not ready or willing. These expressions should be genuine and come from the heart.

- **Respect Individual Preferences:** Respect their individual preferences regarding how they want to communicate and with whom they want to share their feelings.

- **Acknowledge Limitations:** Recognize that not all relationships can be fully reconciled or that some individuals may have difficulty expressing their emotions. The most important thing is to offer support and create space for whatever expression is possible.

Spiritual Support (If Appropriate)

- **Connect with Spiritual Resources:** If the individual is religious or spiritual, connect them with a chaplain, spiritual advisor, or other spiritual resources.

- **Support Spiritual Practices:** Support their spiritual practices, such as prayer, meditation, or rituals.

Facilitating expressions of love and gratitude at the end of life is a precious gift. By offering a safe space, encouraging open communication, and respecting individual wishes, you can help individuals connect with loved ones, express their deepest feelings, and find peace and contentment.

Chapter 13

Memory Making and Legacy Building

Legacy Project

A legacy project is a way for someone to leave a lasting impact and share their story, values, and wisdom with loved ones and future generations. It's a tangible or intangible creation that reflects their life, experiences, and what they hold dear. It can be especially meaningful during end-of-life care, offering a sense of purpose and a way to connect with loved ones even after they're gone.

Benefits of Creating a Legacy Project

Finding Meaning and Purpose:

- **Life Review:** The process of creating a legacy project often involves reflecting on one's life, experiences, and accomplishments. This can help individuals find meaning and purpose in their lives, even as they face death.

- **Sense of Accomplishment:** Completing a legacy project, however small, can provide a sense of accomplishment and fulfillment, counteracting feelings of helplessness or despair.

- **Focus on the Positive:** Creating a legacy project can shift the focus from loss and sadness to appreciation for the positive aspects of life, fostering a sense of gratitude and joy.

Emotional and Spiritual Well-being:

- **Emotional Processing:** The creative process can be a healthy outlet for expressing emotions, such as love, grief, regret, or fear. It can be a way to process these emotions and find peace.

- **Spiritual Connection:** For some, creating a legacy project can be a spiritual experience, allowing them to connect with their beliefs, values, or a sense of something larger than themselves.

- **Reduced Anxiety:** Having a focus and a purpose can reduce anxiety and fear associated with death. It can provide a sense of control during a time when much feels out of control.

Connection and Legacy:

- **Sharing with Loved Ones:** Legacy projects can be a way to connect with loved ones, share memories, and express love and gratitude. It can strengthen bonds and provide comfort to both the creator and the recipient.

- **Leaving a Lasting Impact:** Knowing that their story, wisdom, and values will be preserved can provide a sense of purpose and legacy. It allows individuals to leave a lasting impact on future generations.

- **Preserving Memories:** Legacy projects can be a way to preserve important memories, family history, and cultural heritage.

Personal Growth and Acceptance:

- **Self-Reflection:** The process of creating a legacy project encourages self-reflection and introspection. It can be a way to gain new insights into oneself and one's life.

- **Acceptance:** Working on a legacy project can help individuals come to terms with their mortality and find acceptance in the face of death.

- **Sense of Peace:** Completing a legacy project can bring a sense of peace and closure, allowing individuals to focus on the present moment and cherish their remaining time.

Empowerment and Control:

- **Sense of Agency:** At a time when many things feel beyond control, creating a legacy project can provide a sense of agency and empowerment. It allows individuals to actively participate in shaping their final chapter.

- **Making Choices:** The process of creating a legacy project involves making choices about what to include and how to express it. This can be a way to assert control and autonomy.

In summary, creating a legacy project at the end of life can be a transformative experience. It can help individuals find meaning, connect with loved ones, process emotions, and leave a lasting impact on the world. It's a way to celebrate life, share wisdom, and find peace during a time of significant transition.

Key Characteristics of a Legacy Project

- **Personal:** It's a reflection of the individual's unique life, personality, beliefs, and values.

- **Meaningful:** It holds deep significance for the creator and often for those who will receive it.

- **Lasting:** It's intended to endure beyond the creator's lifetime, ensuring their story and wisdom are preserved.

- **Intentional:** It's a conscious effort to create something that will have a positive impact on others.

Types of Legacy Projects

Legacy projects can take many forms, depending on the individual's interests, skills, and resources.

- **Written**

  - **Memoir or Autobiography:** A written account of their life story, experiences, and lessons learned.

  - **Letters to Loved Ones:** Personal letters expressing love, gratitude, advice, or hopes for the future.

  - **Ethical Will:** A document sharing values, beliefs, and life lessons, rather than just material possessions.

  - **Poetry or Creative Writing:** Expressing thoughts and feelings through creative writing.

  - **Journaling:** Documenting personal reflections, insights, and experiences.

  - **Recipe Book:** Compiling favorite recipes and sharing them with family and friends.

- **Visual**

  - **Photo Albums or Scrapbooks:** Creating visual records of cherished memories and relationships.

- **Video Recordings:** Recording video messages, sharing stories, or documenting life lessons.

- **Artwork:** Creating paintings, drawings, sculptures, or other forms of art.

- **Family Tree:** Creating or updating a family tree, including stories and photos.

- **Audio**

  - **Audio Recordings:** Recording audio messages, sharing stories, or documenting life lessons.

  - **Music Playlists:** Creating playlists of favorite songs that have special meaning.

- **Acts of Service**

  - **Donating to Charity:** Supporting a cause that reflects their values.

  - **Volunteering:** Sharing their time and skills with an organization they care about.

  - **Mentoring:** Sharing their knowledge and experience with others.

- **Other**

    - **Keepsake Box:** Assembling a collection of meaningful items that represent their life.

    - **Planting a Tree:** Planting a tree in their honor.

    - **Creating a Scholarship:** Establishing a scholarship to support future generations.

Why are Legacy Projects Important

- **Preserving Memories:** They help preserve important memories, stories, and family history.

- **Sharing Wisdom:** They offer a way to share life lessons, values, and insights with loved ones.

- **Finding Meaning:** Creating a legacy project can be a meaningful and fulfilling experience, especially during end-of-life care.

- **Connecting with Loved Ones:** They can be a way to connect with loved ones and leave a lasting impact on their lives.

- **Leaving a Legacy:** They provide a tangible or intangible legacy that will endure beyond the creator's lifetime.

Legacy projects are a powerful way for individuals to leave their mark on the world and ensure that their stories and values are remembered and cherished for generations to come. They are a gift to loved ones and a testament to a life well-lived.

Tips for Creating a Legacy

Start Early and Be Patient

- **Time is Precious:** The earlier someone begins thinking about their legacy, the more time and energy they'll have to dedicate to it. Encourage them to start sooner rather than later, even if they don't feel "ready."

- **Pace Yourself:** Creating a legacy doesn't need to be rushed. It's a process of reflection and creation, so allow ample time and avoid pressure.

- **Flexibility:** Be open to evolving ideas. The initial concept for a legacy project might change as the individual reflects and explores different options.

Focus on What Matters Most

- **Values and Beliefs:** What values and beliefs are most important to the individual? What do they want to be remembered for? These questions can help guide the creation process.

- **Key Relationships:** Which relationships are most significant? Is there a particular message they want to convey to specific loved ones?

- **Life Lessons:** What are the most important lessons they've learned in life? What wisdom do they want to share with future generations?

- **Joyful Memories:** What are some of their favorite memories? What moments brought them the most joy and fulfillment?

Choose a Meaningful Format

- **Consider Interests and Skills:** What are the individual's talents and interests? Do they enjoy writing, art, music, or storytelling? The format of the legacy project should align with their strengths and passions.

- **Practical Considerations:** Think about the individual's physical abilities and resources. Choose a format that is realistic and achievable given their current circumstances.

- **Personal Preference:** Ultimately, the best format is the one that resonates most with the individual and allows them to express themselves authentically.

Involve Loved Ones (If Desired)

- **Shared Memories:** Involving family and friends can enrich the legacy project. Sharing stories, photos, and memories can create a more comprehensive and meaningful record.

- **Collaboration:** Family members can assist with the creation process, offering support and encouragement.

- **Passing Down Traditions:** Legacy projects can be a way to pass down family traditions, recipes, or other cultural heritage.

Keep it Manageable

- **Small Gestures, Big Impact:** Legacy projects don't need to be grand or elaborate. Even small gestures, like writing a letter or recording a short video message, can have a significant impact.

- **Break it Down:** Large projects can be broken down into smaller, more manageable tasks. This can make the process less overwhelming.

- **Focus on Progress, Not Perfection:** The goal is to create something meaningful, not perfect. Don't get bogged down in details or strive for flawlessness.

Embrace Imperfection and Authenticity

- **Honesty and Vulnerability:** Encourage the individual to be honest and vulnerable in their expressions. Authenticity is what makes a legacy project truly special.

- **It's Okay to Change:** The content and format of the legacy project can evolve over time. Be flexible and allow for changes as the individual's thoughts and feelings develop.

Don't Pressure

- **Respect Boundaries:** Never pressure someone to create a legacy if they are not interested or don't feel up to it. It's a personal choice, and their wishes should be respected.

- **Offer Support, Not Demands:** Offer your support and encouragement but avoid making demands or setting unrealistic expectations.

Preserve and Share

- **Storage and Distribution:** Think about how the legacy project will be preserved and shared with loved ones. Will it be stored digitally, physically, or both? Who will be responsible for distributing it?

- **Accessibility:** Ensure that the legacy project will be easily accessible to those who are meant to receive it.

Celebrate the Process

- **A Gift of Love:** Creating a legacy is a gift of love and connection. Celebrate the process and acknowledge the individual's efforts.

- **Meaningful Experience:** The act of creating a legacy can be a deeply meaningful and fulfilling experience in itself, regardless of the final product.

Part 4
Supporting the Caregiver

Chapter 14

The Caregiver's Emotional Journey

Caregiving at the end of life is an incredibly demanding experience, both physically and emotionally. It's a time filled with complex emotions, difficult decisions, and profound loss. Caregivers often face a unique set of challenges that can significantly impact their well-being.

Grief and Loss (Anticipatory and Cumulative)

- **Anticipatory Grief:** Caregivers often begin grieving long before the actual death. They grieve the loss of the person as they once were, the loss of shared experiences, and the impending loss of their physical presence.

- **Cumulative Grief:** End-of-life caregiving can involve a series of losses – loss of abilities, loss of independence, loss of cognitive function. These accumulate, creating a heavy burden of grief.

Emotional Rollercoaster

- **Fluctuating Emotions:** Caregivers experience a wide range of emotions, often within a short period. These can include sadness, anger, fear, guilt, anxiety, denial, and even moments of joy and connection.

- **Emotional Exhaustion:** The constant emotional strain can lead to exhaustion, burnout, and difficulty coping.

Stress and Burnout

- **Physical and Emotional Demands:** Caregiving is physically demanding, especially if it involves complex medical needs or around-the-clock care. This, combined with the emotional strain, can lead to caregiver burnout.

- **Lack of Respite:** Caregivers often have little time for themselves or for activities they enjoy. The lack of respite can contribute to stress and resentment.

Guilt and Regret

- **"Not Doing Enough":** Caregivers often struggle with feelings of guilt, believing they are not doing enough for their loved one.

- **Difficult Decisions:** Making difficult decisions about medical care, end-of-life choices, or even basic daily care can lead to regret and self-doubt.

- **Unresolved Issues:** If there are unresolved issues or conflicts in the relationship, these can surface during the caregiving period, leading to guilt and regret.

Anxiety and Fear

- **Fear of the Unknown:** Caregivers often fear the unknown – the dying process, the pain their loved one may experience, and what will happen after death.

- **Anxiety about Care:** They may worry about their ability to provide adequate care and manage complex medical needs.

Isolation and Loneliness

- **Social Withdrawal:** Caregiving can be isolating, limiting social interactions and time with friends and family.

- **Lack of Understanding:** Caregivers may feel that others don't understand what they are going through, leading to feelings of loneliness.

Role Changes and Identity Shifts

- **Shifting Roles:** Caregiving often involves taking on new roles and responsibilities, which can be challenging and overwhelming.

- **Loss of Identity:** Caregivers may feel a loss of their own identity as their lives become consumed by caregiving duties.

Ethical Dilemmas and Decision-Making

- **Difficult Choices:** Caregivers often face difficult ethical dilemmas related to medical treatment, end-of-life decisions, and quality of life.

- **Burden of Responsibility:** The weight of these decisions can be emotionally heavy.

Compassion Fatigue

- **Emotional Depletion:** Constant exposure to suffering and loss can lead to compassion fatigue, a state of emotional and physical exhaustion.

Post-Caregiving Adjustment

- **Grief and Bereavement:** After the death of their loved one, caregivers face the grieving process, which can be intense and prolonged.

- **Readjusting to Life:** Caregivers may struggle to readjust to life after caregiving, finding it difficult to fill the void left by their loved one's absence.

It's important for caregivers to acknowledge these emotional challenges and seek support when needed. This might involve talking to family and friends, joining a support group, seeking professional counseling, or accessing respite care services. Recognizing and addressing these emotional needs is essential for both the caregiver's well-being and the quality of care provided.

Grief

Grief and anticipatory grief are significant challenges for caregivers, and understanding their impact is important for providing compassionate care, both for the person at end-of-life and the caregiver.

Grief in End-of-Life Caregiving

- **It's not just about death:** Grief in this context isn't solely about the loss after death. It encompasses a range of losses experienced *during* the caregiving process:

    o **Loss of the person as they were:** You grieve the changes in your loved one due to illness – physical decline, cognitive changes, personality shifts.

    o **Loss of the relationship as you knew it:** The dynamics of your relationship may shift dramatically, impacting roles, intimacy, and shared activities.

- ○ **Loss of future hopes and dreams:** You may grieve the future you envisioned with your loved one, the experiences you won't share.

  - ○ **Loss of your own life as you knew it:** Caregiving can significantly alter your life, impacting work, social activities, and personal time.

- **It's complex and fluctuating:** Grief can manifest in many ways – sadness, anger, denial, guilt, exhaustion, numbness. These emotions can come in waves, often unpredictable and intense.

Anticipatory Grief

This is a unique form of grief that begins *before* the actual death. It's the emotional process of preparing for the inevitable loss. While painful, it can also be a way to begin the grieving process and find acceptance.

Challenges of Grief and Anticipatory Grief for Caregivers

- **Emotional Burden:** Caring for someone at the end of life is emotionally exhausting. Coupled with your own grief, it can feel overwhelming.

- **Balancing Needs:** You're trying to support your loved one through their own journey while simultaneously processing your own emotions. This can be incredibly difficult to balance.

- **Guilt and Self-Doubt:** You might feel guilty for grieving before the death, or question if you're grieving "correctly." There's no right way to feel.

- **Impact on Caregiving:** Grief can affect your ability to provide care. You may feel less patient, more irritable, or struggle with decision-making.

- **Isolation:** Grief can lead to withdrawal, making it harder to connect with others for support. You might feel like no one understands what you're going through.

Coping Strategies

- **Acknowledge and Validate:** Recognize that your feelings are normal and valid. Don't try to suppress or ignore them.

- **Seek Support:** Talk to trusted friends, family members, or a therapist. Support groups for caregivers can also be incredibly helpful.

- **Self-Care is Crucial:** Prioritize your physical and emotional well-being. This might include exercise, getting enough sleep, eating healthy foods, and engaging in activities you enjoy.

- **Allow Yourself to Grieve:** Don't judge your grief or compare it to others. Allow yourself the time and space to process your emotions.

- **Find Healthy Outlets:** Journaling, creative expression, or spending time in nature can be healthy ways to cope with grief.

- **Professional Help:** If you're struggling to cope, consider seeking professional help from a therapist or counselor.

Remember

- **You are not alone:** Many caregivers experience similar challenges.

- **It's okay to ask for help:** Don't hesitate to reach out for support from family, friends, support groups, or professionals.

- **Your well-being matters:** Taking care of yourself is essential for both your sake and the quality of care you provide.

Grief and anticipatory grief are a natural part of the end-of-life caregiving journey. By acknowledging these challenges and seeking support, you can navigate this difficult time with greater resilience and compassion, both for yourself and your loved one.

Caregiver Burnout

Caregiver burnout during end-of-life care is a very real and serious concern. It's a state of emotional, physical, and mental exhaustion brought on by the prolonged and intense stress of caring for someone nearing the end of their life.

Challenges Caregivers Face

Emotional Exhaustion

- **Constant emotional output:** Caregivers are constantly giving emotionally – providing comfort, reassurance, and support. This can lead to feeling drained and depleted.

- **Witnessing suffering:** Bearing witness to a loved one's pain, decline, and eventual death can be incredibly distressing and emotionally taxing.

- **Complex emotions:** Caregivers often experience a wide range of emotions, including sadness, anger, guilt, fear, and grief, which can be overwhelming and confusing.

Physical Demands

- **Hands-on care:** End-of-life care often involves physically demanding tasks, such as bathing, dressing, feeding, and repositioning.

- **Sleep deprivation:** Caregivers may experience sleep disruptions due to round-the-clock care needs or worry about their loved one.

- **Chronic stress:** The constant stress of caregiving can take a toll on physical health, leading to weakened immune system, aches and pains, and other health problems.

Mental and Cognitive Strain

- **Decision-making:** Caregivers often have to make difficult decisions about medical treatment, end-of-life choices, and daily care, which can be mentally and emotionally draining.

- **Cognitive overload:** Managing medications, appointments, and complex care plans can be cognitively demanding, especially when combined with emotional stress.

- **Loss of focus:** Caregiver burnout can lead to difficulty concentrating, forgetfulness, and impaired judgment.

Social Isolation

- **Limited time for social activities:** Caregiving can consume a significant amount of time, leaving little room for social activities and connections.

- **Withdrawal:** Caregivers may withdraw from social interactions due to exhaustion, lack of time, or feeling misunderstood.

- **Lack of support:** Caregivers may feel isolated if they don't have adequate support from family, friends, or the community.

Role Overload and Loss of Identity

- **Multiple roles:** Caregivers often juggle multiple roles – spouse, parent, child, friend – in addition to their caregiving responsibilities.

- **Loss of self:** Caregivers may lose a sense of their own identity as their lives become consumed by caregiving duties.

Financial Strain

- **Cost of care:** End-of-life care can be expensive, and caregivers may face financial strain due to medical bills, medications, and other expenses.

- **Lost income:** Some caregivers may have to reduce their work hours or quit their jobs to provide care, leading to lost income and financial stress.

Lack of Respite

- **Constant care:** Many caregivers provide care around the clock, leaving little time for rest or breaks.

- **Difficulty asking for help:** Some caregivers may find it difficult to ask for help or may not have access to respite care services.

Consequences of Caregiver Burnout

- **Decreased quality of care:** Burnout can affect a caregiver's ability to provide compassionate and effective care.

- **Health problems:** Caregiver burnout can lead to physical and mental health problems, such as depression, anxiety, weakened immune system, and cardiovascular issues.

- **Relationship strain:** Burnout can strain relationships with family and friends.

- **Increased risk of elder abuse:** In severe cases, caregiver burnout can increase the risk of elder abuse or neglect.

Signs of Caregiver Burnout

Caregiver burnout is a state of emotional, physical, and mental exhaustion caused by the prolonged and intense stress of caring for someone. Recognizing the signs is the first step to getting help. Here are some common symptoms:

Emotional Signs

- **Feeling overwhelmed and constantly stressed:** You feel like you're drowning in your responsibilities and can't keep up.

- **Irritability and impatience:** You snap easily at your loved one or others, even for minor things.

- **Anger and resentment:** You feel resentful towards the person you're caring for, other family members, or even the situation itself.

- **Sadness and hopelessness:** You feel persistently sad, hopeless, or like you're losing your sense of purpose.

- **Anxiety and worry:** You experience excessive worry, nervousness, or fear about the future and your caregiving abilities.

- **Guilt and self-blame:** You feel guilty, even when you're doing your best, and constantly question if you're doing enough.

- **Loss of interest in things you used to enjoy:** You no longer find pleasure in hobbies, social activities, or other things that once brought you joy.

- **Emotional detachment:** You feel emotionally numb or disconnected from the person you're caring for and other loved ones.

- **Difficulty concentrating:** You struggle to focus, make decisions, or remember things.

Physical Signs

- **Changes in sleep patterns:** You experience insomnia, sleeping too much, or restless sleep.

- **Changes in appetite:** You notice significant changes in your eating habits, either eating much more or much less than usual.

- **Fatigue and exhaustion:** You feel constantly tired and drained, even after resting.

- **Physical aches and pains:** You experience unexplained headaches, muscle aches, or other physical discomfort.

- **Weakened immune system:** You get sick more often than usual.

- **Weight changes:** You experience unintentional weight gain or loss.

Behavioral Signs

- **Social withdrawal:** You isolate yourself from friends, family, and social activities.

- **Increased use of alcohol or drugs:** You rely on substances to cope with stress or difficult emotions.

- **Neglecting personal care:** You neglect your own hygiene, grooming, or other basic needs.

- **Making more mistakes than usual:** You find yourself making careless errors in your caregiving tasks.

- **Difficulty setting boundaries:** You struggle to say no to additional responsibilities or requests.

- **Outbursts of anger or frustration:** You may yell, cry, or lash out at others.

Cognitive Signs

- **Forgetfulness:** You become increasingly forgetful about appointments, medications, or other important tasks.

- **Difficulty concentrating:** You struggle to focus, make decisions, or organize your thoughts.

- **Negative thinking:** You have persistent negative thoughts about yourself, the caregiving situation, or the future.

It's important to remember that these signs can vary from person to person. If you're experiencing several of these symptoms, it's a good idea to seek help. Don't hesitate to talk to your doctor, a therapist, or a support group for caregivers. Early intervention can help prevent burnout from becoming overwhelming and impacting your well-being and the quality of care you provide.

It's vital for caregivers to recognize the signs of burnout and seek help early. This might involve:

- **Respite care:** Utilizing respite care services to take breaks from caregiving responsibilities.

- **Support groups:** Joining support groups for caregivers to connect with others who understand their challenges.

- **Counseling or therapy:** Seeking professional help to manage stress, emotions, and coping strategies.

- **Self-care:** Prioritizing self-care activities, such as exercise, healthy eating, relaxation techniques, and hobbies.

- **Setting boundaries:** Learning to say no to additional responsibilities and prioritizing their own needs.

- **Asking for help:** Reaching out to family, friends, or community resources for assistance.

Caregiver burnout is a serious issue, but it's not inevitable. By recognizing the challenges, seeking support, and prioritizing self-care, caregivers can protect their well-being and continue to provide compassionate care for their loved ones.

Strategies for Coping with Burnout

It's essential for caregivers to prioritize their own well-being, especially during the demanding time of end-of-life care. Here are some self-care strategies and coping mechanisms to help deal with caregiver burnout:

Acknowledge and Accept Your Feelings

- **Validate Your Emotions:** Recognize that it's normal to experience a wide range of emotions, including sadness, anger, guilt, fear, and exhaustion. Don't judge yourself for these feelings.

- **Be Honest with Yourself:** Acknowledge the challenges of caregiving and the toll it's taking on you. Don't try to be a "super caregiver" or deny your needs.

- **Seek Professional Help:** If you're struggling to cope with your emotions, don't hesitate to seek professional help from a therapist or counselor.

Prioritize Physical Health

- **Healthy Diet:** Maintain a balanced diet, even when you're short on time. Choose nutritious foods that provide energy and support your physical and emotional well-being.

- **Regular Exercise:** Even short bursts of physical activity can make a difference. Take a walk, stretch, or do some light exercise to boost your mood and reduce stress.

- **Adequate Sleep:** Aim for 7-8 hours of sleep per night. If you're having trouble sleeping, talk to your doctor about strategies to improve your sleep hygiene.

- **Rest and Relaxation:** Schedule regular breaks throughout the day to rest and recharge. Even 15-20 minutes of quiet time can be beneficial.

Engage in Stress-Reducing Activities

- **Mindfulness and Meditation:** Practice mindfulness or meditation techniques to calm your mind and reduce stress.

- **Deep Breathing Exercises:** Deep breathing exercises can help you relax and manage anxiety in the moment.

- **Yoga or Tai Chi:** These practices combine physical movement with mindfulness and can be very effective in reducing stress.

- **Hobbies and Interests:** Make time for activities you enjoy, even if it's just for a short period. Engaging in hobbies can help you relax and recharge.

Seek Support and Connection

- **Talk to Trusted Friends and Family:** Share your feelings and experiences with people you trust. Talking about your challenges can be a great way to release stress and feel supported.

- **Join a Support Group:** Connect with other caregivers who understand what you're going through. Sharing experiences and tips can be incredibly helpful.

- **Respite Care:** Utilize respite care services to take breaks from caregiving responsibilities. Even a few hours of respite can make a big difference.

- **Delegate Tasks:** Don't be afraid to ask for help from family members, friends, or volunteers. Delegate tasks whenever possible to reduce your workload.

Set Boundaries and Say No

- **Prioritize Your Needs:** It's okay to prioritize your own needs and say no to additional responsibilities. You can't pour from an empty cup.

- **Set Limits:** Set limits on what you can do and don't overextend yourself. It's important to be realistic about your capacity.

- **Communicate Your Needs:** Clearly communicate your needs to family members and friends. Let them know what kind of support you need.

Practice Self-Compassion

- **Be Kind to Yourself:** Don't be too hard on yourself. Caregiving is challenging, and it's okay to make mistakes.

- **Acknowledge Your Efforts:** Recognize and appreciate all that you do for your loved one. You are making a difference, even if it doesn't always feel like it.

- **Focus on the Positive:** Try to focus on the positive aspects of caregiving, such as the moments of connection and the love you share.

Plan for the Future

- **Long-Term Care Planning:** If possible, discuss long-term care plans with your loved one and other family members. This can help reduce anxiety about the future.

- **End-of-Life Planning:** Discuss end-of-life wishes with your loved one, including their preferences for medical treatment, pain management, and funeral arrangements.

- **Grief Support:** Consider seeking grief support before your loved one passes away. This can help you prepare for the loss and begin the grieving process.

Remember Your Worth

- **You Are Making a Difference:** You are providing invaluable care and support to your loved one. Your efforts are making a difference, even if you don't always see it.

- **You Are Not Alone:** Many caregivers are going through similar challenges. Reach out for support and connect with others who understand.

- **You Deserve Support:** You deserve to be supported and cared for, just as you are caring for your loved one.

By implementing these self-care strategies and coping mechanisms, caregivers can reduce their risk of burnout and continue to provide compassionate care while prioritizing their own well-being. Remember, taking care of yourself is not selfish; it's essential for both your sake and the quality of care you provide.

Chapter 15

Managing Family Dynamics

Navigating Family Conflicts, Disagreements, and Differing Opinions Regarding End-of-Life Care

End-of-life caregiving is a deeply challenging yet profoundly meaningful experience. It's a time when families often come together to support a loved one through their final journey. However, even in the most loving families, disagreements, differing opinions, and conflicts can arise regarding end-of-life care. These conflicts can add significant stress to an already difficult situation, impacting both the quality of care provided and the emotional well-being of everyone involved. This comprehensive article explores the common sources of family conflict in end-of-life care, offers strategies for navigating these challenges, and emphasizes the importance of prioritizing the well-being of both the dying individual and the caregivers.

Understanding the Landscape of Conflict

End-of-life care decisions are rarely simple. They often involve complex medical choices, ethical considerations, deeply held personal beliefs, and the emotional weight of impending loss. It's no surprise that families, each with their own unique perspectives and experiences, may find themselves at odds. Understanding the common roots of these conflicts is the first step towards navigating them effectively.

Common Sources of Conflict

- **Differing Values and Beliefs:** Families are comprised of individuals with diverse values, cultural backgrounds, religious beliefs, and personal philosophies. These differences can significantly influence perspectives on medical interventions, the definition of quality of life, and approaches to death and dying. For example, some family members may prioritize prolonging life at all costs, while others may emphasize comfort and quality of remaining time.

- **Emotional Responses to Grief and Loss:** Grief is a complex and highly personal experience. The impending loss of a loved one can trigger a range of powerful emotions – fear, sadness, anger, denial, guilt – that can influence decision-making and lead to disagreements. Family members may be at different stages of the grieving process, further complicating communication.

- **Past Family Dynamics and Unresolved Conflicts:** Pre-existing family dynamics, including long-standing rivalries, communication patterns, and unresolved

315

conflicts, can resurface and intensify during times of stress. Old wounds can be reopened, making it difficult to address current issues constructively.

- **Lack of Information or Misunderstandings:** Misunderstandings about the loved one's medical condition, prognosis, or treatment options can contribute to conflict. Lack of clear and consistent communication from healthcare providers can exacerbate these misunderstandings.

- **Control Issues and Power Struggles:** End-of-life care decisions can evoke feelings of powerlessness. Some family members may attempt to assert control over the situation, leading to power struggles and conflict. This can be particularly challenging when there is a designated decision-maker (e.g., healthcare proxy) whose authority is being questioned.

- **Financial Concerns:** The costs associated with end-of-life care can be substantial, and financial concerns can add another layer of complexity to family discussions. Disagreements may arise regarding the allocation of resources or the potential financial burden on individual family members.

- **Differing Perceptions of "Best Interests":** What constitutes "best interests" for the dying individual can be subjective and open to interpretation. Family members may have different ideas about what constitutes a good quality of life or what level of medical intervention is appropriate, leading to conflict.

- **Caregiver Stress and Burnout:** Caregiving is a demanding role, and caregivers often experience significant stress and burnout. This can lead to increased irritability, reduced patience, and difficulty communicating effectively, contributing to family conflict.

Strategies for Navigating Conflict

While conflict is often unavoidable, it can be managed constructively. The following strategies can help families navigate disagreements and make decisions collaboratively:

- **Proactive Communication and Planning:** Ideally, discussions about end-of-life care preferences should begin *before* a crisis occurs. This allows for calmer, more thoughtful conversations. Encourage the loved one to complete advance directives (living will, durable power of attorney for healthcare), which can provide invaluable guidance when they are no longer able to express their wishes. Hold regular family meetings to discuss care plans, address concerns, and ensure everyone is on the same page.

- **Active Listening and Empathy:** Encourage everyone to practice active listening. This means truly hearing and trying to understand each other's perspectives, even if they disagree. Empathy is key – acknowledge and validate each other's feelings, recognizing that everyone is likely experiencing a range of difficult emotions.

- **Respectful Communication:** Insist on respectful communication. Discourage blaming, name-calling, interrupting, or other forms of disrespectful behavior. Encourage family members to express their opinions calmly and respectfully, focusing on "I" statements rather than accusatory "you" statements.

- **Focus on the Loved One's Best Interests:** Remind everyone that the primary focus should be the well-being and comfort of the individual receiving care. Decisions should be guided by their wishes and preferences, as expressed in advance directives or through conversations.

- **Identify Common Ground and Shared Goals:** Even when there are disagreements, there are often areas of common ground. Focus on these shared goals and use them as a starting point for further discussion and compromise.

- **Seek Mediation or Professional Facilitation:** If conflicts are escalating or proving difficult to resolve within the family, consider involving a neutral third party. A professional mediator, counselor, or chaplain can help facilitate communication and guide the discussion towards a resolution.

- **Involve the Healthcare Team:** The healthcare team, including doctors, nurses, and social workers, can play a vital role in resolving family conflicts. They can provide accurate information about the loved one's condition, explain treatment options, and help facilitate communication between family members. They can also offer support and guidance on ethical dilemmas.

- **Acknowledge and Manage Emotions:** Recognize that everyone is likely experiencing a range of difficult emotions, including grief, fear, and anxiety. Acknowledge these emotions and create space for family members to express them in a healthy way. Encourage self-care and offer support to those who are struggling.

- **Compromise and Flexibility:** Compromise is often necessary to reach a consensus. Encourage family members to be flexible and willing to consider alternative solutions. It may not be possible for everyone to get exactly what they want but finding a solution that everyone can live with is essential.

- **Documentation and Record Keeping:** Keep clear and detailed records of family discussions, decisions made, and any agreements reached. This can help prevent misunderstandings and ensure that everyone is on the same page.

- **Respect Boundaries and Individual Roles:** Recognize that each family member has a unique role to play. Respect individual boundaries and avoid assigning roles or responsibilities that are unwanted or overwhelming.

- **Know When to Step Back:** Sometimes, despite everyone's best efforts, it may not be possible to fully resolve all conflicts. It's important to recognize when to step back and accept that some disagreements may remain. Focus on providing comfort and support to the loved one, even if family members are not in complete agreement.

When Agreement Can't Be Reached

In some situations, despite all efforts, families may not be able to reach a unanimous agreement. In these cases, the following strategies may be necessary:

- **Majority Rule (with Caution):** In some cases, a majority vote may be necessary to make decisions. However, this approach should be used cautiously and with sensitivity, as it can leave some family members feeling unheard or disregarded.

- **Designated Decision-Maker:** If the loved one has designated a healthcare proxy or durable power of attorney for healthcare, that individual has the legal authority to make decisions on their behalf. Other family members should respect this designation, even if they disagree with the decisions being made.

- **Ethics Committee Consultation:** Hospitals and healthcare facilities often have ethics committees that can provide guidance on complex ethical dilemmas. These committees can help families explore different options and make decisions that are consistent with the loved one's values and wishes.

- **Court Intervention (as a Last Resort):** In rare cases, if there is a legal dispute about who has the authority to make medical decisions, it may be necessary to seek court intervention. However, this should be considered a last resort, as it can be costly, time-consuming, and emotionally draining.

Self-Care for Caregivers

Navigating family conflicts during end-of-life care can be incredibly stressful for caregivers. It's essential to prioritize self-care and seek support when needed. This might involve:

- **Setting Boundaries:** It's important for caregivers to set boundaries and protect their own well-being. Avoid getting drawn into every argument or taking responsibility for resolving all conflicts.

- **Seeking Support:** Talk to trusted friends, family members, or a therapist about the stress and challenges you're facing. Support groups for caregivers can also be incredibly helpful.

- **Respite Care:** Utilize respite care services to take breaks from caregiving responsibilities.

Even a few hours of respite can make a big difference.

- **Practicing Self-Compassion:** Be kind to yourself and recognize that you are doing the best you can under difficult circumstances.

The Importance of Prioritizing the Dying Individual

Throughout the process of navigating family conflicts, it's important to remember that the primary focus should always be the well-being and comfort of the individual receiving care. Their wishes and preferences should be central to all discussions and decisions. Even when family members disagree, they should strive to create a peaceful and supportive environment

Facilitating Communication and Promoting Understanding When Disagreements and Conflicts Arise

Understanding the Roots of Conflict

End-of-life care decisions are rarely straightforward. They involve a complex interplay of medical factors, personal values, religious beliefs, emotional responses to grief, and pre-existing family dynamics. Understanding the common sources of conflict is crucial for developing effective strategies for resolution.

Common Triggers for Family Disagreements

- **Differing Values and Beliefs:** Families are composed of individuals with diverse backgrounds, values, religious beliefs, and cultural norms. These differences can significantly influence perspectives on medical interventions, the definition of quality of life, and approaches to death and dying. For example, some family members may prioritize prolonging life through aggressive treatment, while others may emphasize comfort and palliative care.

- **Emotional Responses to Grief and Loss:** Grief is a complex and highly personal experience. The impending loss of a loved one can trigger a range of powerful emotions – fear, sadness, anger, denial, guilt – that can influence decision-making and lead to disagreements. Family members may be at different stages of the grieving process, further complicating communication.

- **Past Family Dynamics and Unresolved Conflicts:** Long-standing family rivalries, communication patterns, and unresolved conflicts can resurface and intensify during times of stress. Old wounds can be reopened, making it difficult to address current issues constructively.

- **Lack of Information or Misunderstandings:** Misunderstandings about the loved one's medical condition, prognosis, or treatment options can contribute to conflict. Lack of clear and consistent communication from healthcare providers can exacerbate these misunderstandings.

- **Control Issues and Power Struggles:** End-of-life care decisions can evoke feelings of powerlessness. Some family members may attempt to assert control over the situation, leading to power struggles and conflict. This can be particularly challenging when there is a designated decision-maker (e.g., healthcare proxy) whose authority is being questioned.

- **Financial Concerns:** The costs associated with end-of-life care can be substantial, and financial concerns can add another layer of complexity to family discussions. Disagreements may arise regarding the allocation of resources or the potential financial burden on individual family members.

- **Differing Perceptions of "Best Interests":** What constitutes "best interests" for the dying individual can be subjective and open to interpretation. Family members may have different ideas about what constitutes a good quality of life or what level of medical intervention is appropriate, leading to conflict.

- **Caregiver Stress and Burnout:** Caregiving is a demanding role, and caregivers often experience significant stress and burnout. This can lead to increased irritability, reduced patience, and difficulty communicating effectively, contributing to family conflict.

Strategies for Facilitating Communication and Promoting Understanding

Navigating family disagreements requires a proactive and compassionate approach. The following strategies can help families communicate more effectively and work towards shared understanding:

- **Proactive Communication and Advance Care Planning:** Ideally, discussions about end-of-life care preferences should begin *before* a crisis occurs. This allows for calmer, more thoughtful conversations. Encourage the loved one to complete advance directives (living will, durable power of attorney for healthcare), which can provide invaluable guidance when they are no longer able to express their wishes. Hold regular family meetings to discuss care plans, address concerns, and ensure everyone is on the same page.

- **Create a Safe and Supportive Environment:** Establish a safe and respectful environment for communication. Emphasize that everyone's opinions and feelings are valued, and that open and honest dialogue is essential. Choose a quiet and private space where family members can feel comfortable sharing their thoughts.

- **Active Listening and Empathy:** Encourage everyone to practice active listening. This means truly hearing and trying to understand each other's perspectives, even if they disagree. Empathy is key – acknowledge and validate each other's feelings, recognizing that everyone is likely experiencing a range of difficult emotions. Try to understand the underlying concerns and motivations behind each person's perspective.

- **Focus on Shared Goals and Values:** Even when there are disagreements, there are often shared goals and values. Focus on these commonalities and use them as a foundation for further discussion. For example, everyone likely wants the loved one to be comfortable and receive the best possible care.

- **Seek Mediation or Professional Facilitation:** If conflicts are escalating or proving difficult to resolve within the family, consider involving a neutral third party. A professional mediator, counselor, or chaplain can help facilitate communication, guide the discussion towards a resolution, and offer an objective perspective.

- **Involve the Healthcare Team:** The healthcare team, including doctors, nurses, and social workers, can play a vital role in resolving family conflicts. They can provide accurate information about the loved one's condition, explain treatment options, and help facilitate communication between family members. They can also offer support and guidance on ethical dilemmas.

- **Acknowledge and Manage Emotions:** Recognize that everyone is likely experiencing a range of difficult emotions, including grief, fear, and anxiety. Acknowledge these emotions and create space for family members to express them in a healthy way. Encourage self-care and offer support to those who are struggling.

- **Promote Understanding of Medical Information:** Ensure that everyone has access to clear and accurate information about the loved one's medical condition, prognosis, and treatment options. Encourage family members to ask questions and seek clarification from healthcare providers. Translate complex medical jargon into easily understandable language.

- **Compromise and Flexibility:** Compromise is often necessary to reach a consensus. Encourage family members to be flexible and willing to consider alternative solutions. It may not be possible for everyone to get exactly what they want but finding a solution that everyone can live with is essential.

- **Documentation and Record Keeping:** Keep clear and detailed records of family discussions, decisions made, and any agreements reached. This can help prevent misunderstandings and ensure that everyone is on the same page. Document the loved one's wishes and preferences as clearly as possible.

- **Respect Boundaries and Individual Roles:** Recognize that each family member has a unique role to play. Respect individual boundaries and avoid assigning roles or responsibilities that are unwanted or overwhelming. Allow each person to contribute in a way that feels comfortable and meaningful to them.

- **Focus on the Present Moment:** During times of stress, it's easy to get caught up in worries about the future. Encourage family members to focus on the present moment and cherish the time they have together.

- **Know When to Step Back:** Sometimes, despite everyone's best efforts, it may not be possible to fully resolve all conflicts. It's important to recognize when to step back and accept that some disagreements may remain. Focus on providing comfort and support to the loved one, even if family members are not in complete agreement.

When Agreement Can't Be Reached

In some situations, despite all efforts, families may not be able to reach a unanimous agreement. In these cases, the following strategies may be necessary:

- **Majority Rule (with Caution):** In some cases, a majority vote may be necessary to make decisions. However, this approach should be used cautiously and with sensitivity, as it can leave some family members feeling unheard or disregarded. It's important to ensure that everyone has had a chance to express their views before resorting to a vote.

- **Designated Decision-Maker:** If the loved one has designated a healthcare proxy or durable power of attorney for healthcare, that individual has the legal authority to make decisions on their behalf. Other family members should respect this designation, even if they disagree with the decisions being made. The designated decision-maker should strive to act in accordance with the loved one's wishes and values, as expressed in advance directives or through conversations.

- **Ethics Committee Consultation:** Hospitals and healthcare facilities often have ethics committees that can provide guidance on complex ethical dilemmas. These committees can help families explore different options and make decisions that are consistent with the loved one's values and wishes. They can also offer a neutral perspective and facilitate discussions about challenging ethical issues.

- **Court Intervention (as a Last Resort):** In rare cases, if there is a legal dispute about who has the authority to make medical decisions, it may be necessary to seek court intervention. However, this should be considered a last resort, as it can be costly, time-consuming, and emotionally draining.

Self-Care for Caregivers

Navigating family conflicts during end-of-life care can be incredibly stressful for caregivers. It's essential to prioritize self-care and seek support when needed. This might involve:

- **Setting Boundaries:** It's important for caregivers to set boundaries and protect their own well-being. Avoid getting drawn into every argument or taking responsibility for resolving all conflicts. It's okay to step away from difficult conversations when needed.

- **Seeking Support:** Talk to trusted friends, family members, or a therapist about the stress and challenges you

Chapter 16

The Importance of Respite Care

The Need for Breaks and Respite Care

The relentless demands of end-of-life care can take a significant toll, impacting the caregiver's well-being and, ultimately, the quality of care they can provide. We will explore the need for caregivers to prioritize their own well-being by taking regular breaks and utilizing respite care services and delve into the benefits of respite, and practical strategies for caregivers to access and utilize these essential resources.

The Importance of Breaks and Respite Care

Breaks and respite care are not luxuries for caregivers; they are essential for maintaining well-being and preventing burnout. Respite care provides temporary relief from caregiving responsibilities, allowing caregivers to:

- **Recharge and Rejuvenate:** Time away from caregiving allows caregivers to rest, relax, and engage in activities they enjoy. This helps them recharge emotionally and physically.

- **Reduce Stress and Improve Mood:** Regular breaks can significantly reduce stress levels, improve mood, and enhance overall well-being.

- **Maintain Physical and Mental Health:** Respite care helps prevent the physical and mental health problems associated with caregiver burnout.

- **Reconnect with Others:** Time away from caregiving allows caregivers to reconnect with friends, family, and social activities, reducing feelings of isolation.

- **Attend to Personal Needs:** Caregivers can use respite time to attend to their own medical appointments, errands, and other personal needs that may have been neglected.

- **Improve Caregiving Skills:** Taking breaks can actually enhance caregiving skills by preventing burnout and allowing caregivers to return to their responsibilities feeling refreshed and more focused.

Types of Respite Care

Respite care can be provided in various settings and formats, depending on the caregiver's needs and preferences:

- **In-Home Respite:** A trained caregiver comes to the home to provide care for the loved one, allowing the primary caregiver to take a break.

- **Adult Day Care:** The loved one attends a day program that provides social activities, meals, and supervision, giving the caregiver some time off.

- **Short-Term Residential Care:** The loved one stays in a residential facility for a short period, such as a few days or weeks, providing the caregiver with extended respite.

- **Companion Care:** A companion provides non-medical support, such as companionship, errands, or light housekeeping, freeing up the caregiver's time.

- **Volunteer Respite:** Volunteers may offer respite care services, often through community organizations or faith-based groups.

Strategies for Accessing and Utilizing Respite Care

Many caregivers hesitate to seek respite care, feeling guilty or believing they can manage everything on their own. However, it's crucial to recognize the importance of self-care and overcome these barriers. Here are some strategies for accessing and utilizing respite care:

- **Recognize the Need:** Acknowledge that taking breaks is essential, not selfish. Pay attention to the signs of caregiver burnout and don't wait until you're completely overwhelmed to seek help.

- **Talk to Your Loved One:** Discuss the possibility of respite care with your loved one. Explain that it will benefit both of you and allow you to provide better care.

- **Contact Your Local Area Agency on Aging:** These agencies can provide information about respite care services in your community, including funding options and eligibility requirements.

- **Check with Your Insurance Provider:** Some insurance plans may cover a portion of the cost of respite care. Contact your insurance provider to inquire about your coverage.

- **Explore Community Resources:** Many community organizations, such as senior centers, hospitals, and volunteer groups, offer respite care services.

- **Network with Other Caregivers:** Connect with other caregivers in your area through support groups or online forums. They can share their experiences and provide valuable tips on accessing respite care.

- **Plan Ahead:** Don't wait until you're in crisis to look for respite care. Start researching options and making arrangements in advance.

- **Be Specific About Your Needs:** When requesting respite care, be clear about your needs and the type of care your loved one requires.

- **Don't Feel Guilty:** Remember that taking breaks is essential for your well-being and allows you to be a more effective caregiver. Don't feel guilty about taking time for yourself.

Creating a Support System

In addition to formal respite care, building a strong support system can be invaluable for caregivers. This might include:

- **Family and Friends:** Reach out to family members and friends for help with specific tasks, such as errands, transportation, or light housekeeping.

- **Neighbors:** Talk to your neighbors about your caregiving responsibilities. They may be willing to offer assistance with small tasks or provide companionship for your loved one.

- **Faith-Based Communities:** If you are involved in a faith-based community, reach out to your church, synagogue, or other religious organization for support.

- **Online Support Groups:** Connect with other caregivers online through support groups or forums. Sharing experiences and tips can be incredibly helpful.

Resources for Caregivers

Finding respite care can feel overwhelming, but many resources are available to help caregivers access this crucial support. Here's a breakdown of places to look:

National Organizations

- **ARCH National Respite Network and Resource Center:** (archrespite.org) This is a great starting point. ARCH provides a national respite locator, information on funding, and resources for caregivers.

- **The National Respite Coalition:** (nationalrespite.org) Advocates for respite care and offers resources and information.

- **Family Caregiver Alliance (FCA):** (caregiver.org) Provides information, resources, and support for family caregivers, including help with finding respite care. They often have state-specific resources.

- **AARP (American Association of Retired Persons):** (aarp.org) While not solely focused on respite, AARP offers resources and information on caregiving, including finding help and support.

Local and Regional Resources

- **Your Local Area Agency on Aging (AAA):** This is often the best place to start. AAAs connect seniors and their caregivers with local resources, including respite care options, funding assistance, and other support services. You can typically find your local AAA by searching online for "[your county/city] Area Agency on Aging."

- **Your State's Department of Aging or Human Services:** These agencies often have programs and resources related to caregiving and respite.

- **Hospice and Palliative Care Organizations:** Even if your loved one isn't currently in hospice, these organizations can sometimes offer information about respite resources in your community.

- **Hospitals and Healthcare Systems:** Many hospitals have social work departments that can assist with finding community resources, including respite care.

- **Senior Centers:** Local senior centers often provide information about respite options and may even offer some respite services themselves, such as adult day care.

- **Disability-Specific Organizations:** If your loved one has a specific disability (e.g., Alzheimer's, Parkinson's), organizations related to that condition may have respite resources.

- **Community Organizations:** Local churches, synagogues, community centers, and volunteer organizations may offer respite programs or connect you with volunteers who can provide care.

Online Search Strategies

- **Search for "respite care [your city/state]" or "caregiver support [your city/state]"**: This will help you find local resources.

- **Look for "respite care grants" or "respite care assistance"**: Many organizations offer financial assistance for respite care.

Other Tips for Finding Respite Care

- **Talk to your loved one's doctor or other healthcare providers:** They may be able to recommend respite care providers or connect you with resources.

- **Ask friends, family, and neighbors for recommendations:** Personal referrals can be valuable.

- **Check online reviews and testimonials:** Read reviews of respite care providers to get a sense of their quality of service.

- **Interview potential respite care providers:** Ask about their experience, qualifications, and fees. Make sure you feel comfortable with them caring for your loved one.

- **Don't be afraid to ask for help:** Many caregivers hesitate to seek respite care, but it's important to remember that taking care of yourself is essential for providing good care to your loved one.

Remember: Finding the right respite care takes time and effort. Be patient and persistent, and don't give up. The support you receive will be invaluable.

Prioritizing Self-Care

Self-care is not a luxury for caregivers; it's a necessity. In addition to taking breaks and utilizing respite care, caregivers should prioritize the following self-care practices:

- **Healthy Diet:** Maintain a balanced diet, even when you're short on time.

- **Regular Exercise:** Even short bursts of physical activity can make a difference.

- **Adequate Sleep:** Aim for 7-8 hours of sleep per night.

- **Stress Management Techniques:** Practice mindfulness, meditation, deep breathing exercises, or other stress-reducing techniques.

- **Hobbies and Interests:** Make time for activities you enjoy, even if it's just for a short period.

- **Social Connection:** Stay connected with friends and family.

- **Professional Help:** Don't hesitate to seek professional help from a therapist or counselor if you're struggling to cope.

Remember

Caregiving is a marathon, not a sprint. Taking breaks and utilizing respite care is not a sign of weakness; it's a sign of strength and self-awareness. By prioritizing your own well-being, you can ensure that you are able to provide the best possible care for your loved one while also preserving your own health and quality of life. You are not alone in this journey, and there are resources available to support you. Don't hesitate to reach out and ask for help. You deserve it.

Chapter 17

Grief and Bereavement

Grief After Losing a Loved One

When the caregiving journey ends with the passing of a loved one, another journey begins: the journey of grief. Grief is not a linear process with predictable stages; it's a complex, deeply personal, and often tumultuous experience that can profoundly impact every aspect of a caregiver's life.

Understanding the Landscape of Grief

Grief is the natural response to loss, and the death of a loved one is one of life's most significant losses.

It's not simply an emotion; it's a multifaceted experience that encompasses physical, emotional, cognitive, social, and spiritual dimensions. It's important to understand that grief is not a disease to be cured, but a human process to be navigated.

The Multifaceted Nature of Grief

- **Emotional Rollercoaster:** Grief can trigger a wide range of intense emotions, including sadness, anger, guilt, denial, confusion, disbelief, relief, and even moments of joy intertwined with sorrow. These emotions can fluctuate unpredictably, sometimes within the same day.

- **Physical Manifestations:** Grief can manifest physically in various ways, such as fatigue, changes in appetite and sleep patterns, headaches, muscle aches, digestive problems, weakened immune system, and even heart palpitations.

- **Cognitive Impact:** Grief can affect cognitive functions, leading to difficulty concentrating, memory problems, forgetfulness, and a sense of detachment or "brain fog."

- **Social Changes:** Grief can impact social interactions. Some individuals may withdraw from social connections, while others may seek solace in the company of loved ones. Relationships can be strained or strengthened during this time.

- **Spiritual Exploration:** Grief can prompt individuals to question their beliefs about life, death, and the afterlife. Some may find comfort in their faith, while others may struggle with spiritual doubts.

Beyond the "Stages"

While the five stages of grief (denial, anger, bargaining, depression, acceptance) popularized by

Elisabeth Kübler-Ross are widely recognized, it's crucial to understand that grief is not a linear progression through these stages. Individuals may experience these stages in different orders, skip some stages altogether, or revisit certain stages multiple times. Grief is a unique and individual experience, and there is no "right" way to grieve.

Types of Grief

Grief can manifest in various forms, each with its own unique characteristics:

- **Normal Grief:** This encompasses the typical emotional, physical, and cognitive responses to loss. While intense, these responses tend to lessen over time.

- **Complicated Grief:** This is a prolonged and intense form of grief that interferes with daily life. Individuals may experience persistent feelings of sadness, anger, or guilt, difficulty accepting the death, and an inability to move forward.

- **Anticipatory Grief:** This begins *before* the actual death, often during a prolonged illness. It allows individuals to begin processing the impending loss, but it can also be emotionally draining.

- **Disenfranchised Grief:** This type of grief is not openly acknowledged or socially supported. Examples include the loss of a pet or a miscarriage.

- **Cumulative Grief:** This occurs when multiple losses occur in a short period, compounding the grieving process.

Challenges Specific to Caregiver Grief

Caregivers often face a unique set of challenges in their grieving process:

- **Loss of Role and Purpose:** Caregiving often becomes a central part of a caregiver's identity. After the death of their loved one, they may experience a loss of role and purpose, leading to feelings of emptiness and disorientation.

- **Exhaustion and Burnout:** Caregivers are often physically and emotionally exhausted from the demands of caregiving. This can make it more difficult to cope with grief.

- **Guilt and Regret:** Caregivers may experience guilt and regret, wondering if they could have done more or questioning their decisions.

- **Delayed Grief:** Sometimes, caregivers may postpone their own grieving process while focusing on the needs of the dying individual or other family members. This delayed grief can surface later, often with greater intensity.

- **Ambiguous Loss:** In some cases, the loss may be ambiguous, such as when a loved one is missing or has a condition like dementia that gradually erodes their identity. This type of loss can be particularly challenging to grieve.

Navigating the Grief Journey

There is no roadmap for navigating grief, but there are strategies that can help individuals cope and heal:

- **Allow Yourself to Feel:** Acknowledge and validate your emotions. Don't try to suppress or ignore them. Allow yourself to cry, express anger, or feel sadness.

- **Seek Support:** Connect with trusted friends, family members, or a support group. Sharing your feelings with others who understand can be incredibly helpful.

- **Professional Help:** Consider seeking professional help from a therapist or counselor. A therapist can provide a safe space to process your grief and develop coping strategies.

- **Self-Care is Essential:** Prioritize your physical and emotional well-being. Eat nutritious foods, get regular exercise, and aim for adequate sleep. Engage in activities you enjoy, even if you don't feel like it.

- **Be Patient with Yourself:** Grief takes time. Be patient with yourself and allow yourself to grieve at your own pace. Don't compare your experience to others.

- **Honor Your Loved One's Memory:** Find ways to honor the memory of your loved one. This might involve creating a memory book, sharing stories, or engaging in activities that were meaningful to them.

- **Find Meaning and Purpose:** Over time, you may begin to find new meaning and purpose in your life. This might involve pursuing new interests, volunteering, or connecting with your community.

- **Embrace the Journey:** Grief is a journey, not a destination. There will be ups and downs, good days and bad days. Embrace the journey and allow yourself to heal.

Supporting a Grieving Caregiver

If you know someone who is grieving the loss of a loved one after a period of caregiving, here are some ways you can offer support:

- **Be Present:** Simply being present and offering your support can be incredibly helpful. Listen without judgment and offer comfort without trying to "fix" their grief.

- **Offer Practical Help:** Offer to help with practical tasks, such as errands, cooking, or childcare.

- **Acknowledge Their Loss:** Acknowledge their loss and express your condolences. Avoid offering platitudes or minimizing their pain.

- **Check In Regularly:** Check in with them regularly, even if it's just to say hello and let them know you're thinking of them.

- **Encourage Professional Help:** Encourage them to seek professional help if they are struggling to cope.

- **Be Patient:** Grief takes time. Be patient with them and allow them to grieve at their own pace.

Grief is a universal human experience, but it is also a deeply personal one. There is no right or wrong way to grieve, and there is no timeline for healing. By understanding the complexities of grief, offering support, and prioritizing self-care, caregivers and their loved ones can navigate this challenging journey toward healing and acceptance.

Resources

The Many Faces of Grief

Grief manifests differently in each individual, but some common experiences include:

- **Emotional Storm:** A whirlwind of emotions, including sadness, anger, guilt, denial, confusion, disbelief, relief, and even joy intertwined with sorrow, is common. These emotions can shift rapidly and unexpectedly.

- **Physical Echoes:** Grief can manifest physically through fatigue, changes in appetite and sleep patterns, headaches, muscle aches, digestive issues, a weakened immune system, and even heart palpitations.

- **Cognitive Clouding:** Difficulty concentrating, memory problems, forgetfulness, a sense of detachment, and "brain fog" are common cognitive effects of grief.

- **Social Shifts:** Grief can impact social interactions, leading to withdrawal or a strong desire for connection. Relationships can be strained or strengthened during this time.

- **Spiritual Searching:** Grief can prompt existential questions about life, death, and the afterlife. Some may find solace in faith, while others may grapple with spiritual doubts.

Resources for Grief Support

Navigating grief is a challenging journey, but numerous resources are available to provide support and guidance:

National Organizations

- **The National Alliance for Grieving Children:** (childrengrieve.org) Offers resources specifically for children and teens experiencing grief, including support groups, camps, and educational materials.

- **The Dougy Center:** (dougy.org) Provides support groups and resources for children, teens, young adults, and their families grieving a death.

- **The Compassionate Friends:** (compassionatefriends.org) Offers peer support groups for parents who have lost a child.

- **The Tragedy Assistance Program for Survivors (TAPS):** (taps.org) Provides support and resources for those grieving the loss of a military loved one.

- **The National Hospice and Palliative Care Organization (NHPCO):** (nhpco.org) Offers resources on grief and bereavement, including a helpline and online information.

- **The Center for Loss and Life Transition:** (centerforloss.com) Provides resources, books, and workshops on grief and loss.

- **HelpGuide.org:** (helpguide.org) Offers comprehensive articles on coping with grief and loss.

- **AARP (American Association of Retired Persons):** (aarp.org) While not solely focused on grief, AARP provides resources and information on caregiving and loss.

Local Resources

- **Hospice Organizations:** Most hospice organizations offer bereavement services to families and the community, even if the deceased was not a hospice patient. These services may include support groups, individual counseling, and memorial services.

- **Mental Health Professionals:** Therapists and counselors specializing in grief and loss can provide individual or family therapy.

- **Places of Worship:** Many religious communities offer grief support groups or individual counseling through their clergy or lay leaders.

- **Community Centers:** Some community centers offer grief support groups or workshops.

- **Area Agencies on Aging:** These agencies connect seniors and their caregivers with local resources, including grief support services.

- **Local Bereavement Centers:** Many communities have dedicated bereavement centers offering support groups, workshops, and individual counseling.

Online Resources

- **Grief websites and forums:** Websites like What's Your Grief (whatsyourgrief.com), Modern Loss (modernloss.com), and Grief.com offer articles, personal stories, and online communities for those grieving.

- **Online support groups:** Many online platforms host grief support groups, allowing connection with others who have experienced similar losses.

Finding the Right Support

Choosing the right grief support is a personal decision. Consider the following:

- **Type of Loss:** Some resources are tailored to specific losses, such as the death of a child or a spouse.

- **Personal Preferences:** Some prefer individual counseling, while others find support groups more helpful.

- **Accessibility:** Consider location, cost, and scheduling when choosing resources.

- **Explore Options:** Don't hesitate to try different resources until finding what feels right.

Supporting a Grieving Caregiver

If you know someone grieving after caregiving, offer your support:

- **Be Present:** Offer your presence and listen without judgment.

- **Offer Practical Help:** Assist with errands, meals, or childcare.

- **Acknowledge Their Loss:** Express condolences and acknowledge their pain.

- **Check In Regularly:** Stay in touch and offer ongoing support.

- **Encourage Professional Help:** Suggest professional counseling if they are struggling.

- **Be Patient:** Grief takes time. Be patient and understanding.

Remember: Grief is a unique journey. There's no right or wrong way to grieve, and there's no set timeline for healing. Be kind to yourself and allow yourself the time and space you need. Support is available; don't hesitate to reach out. You don't have to navigate this alone.

Part 5

Practical Considerations and Resources

Chapter 18

Hospice and Palliative Care

Embracing Comfort and Dignity – The Benefits of Hospice and Palliative Care

In this landscape of uncertainty, hospice and palliative care emerge as beacons of hope, offering a holistic approach to care that prioritizes quality of life, comfort, and dignity. In this section we will delve into the distinct yet interconnected roles of hospice and palliative care, exploring their numerous benefits for both patients and their families, and highlighting how these specialized care models can enhance the end-of-life experience.

Hospice vs. Palliative Care

While often used interchangeably, hospice and palliative care are distinct yet complementary approaches to care. Understanding their unique roles is crucial for making informed decisions about end-of-life care.

- **Palliative Care:** Palliative care focuses on providing relief from the symptoms and stress of a serious illness, regardless of the diagnosis or stage of the illness. It aims to improve the quality of life for both the patient and their family by addressing physical, emotional, social, and spiritual needs. Palliative care can be provided alongside curative treatment.

- **Hospice Care:** Hospice care is a specialized type of palliative care for individuals with a terminal illness and a life expectancy of six months or less, if the illness runs its normal course. It emphasizes comfort, dignity, and quality of life, rather than curative treatment. Hospice focuses on holistic care, addressing the physical, emotional, social, and spiritual needs of the patient and their family during the final stages of life.

The Interconnectedness of Hospice and Palliative Care

Although distinct, hospice and palliative care share a common philosophy: to enhance quality of life and provide compassionate care to individuals facing serious illness. Palliative care can be offered at any stage of a serious illness, while hospice is specifically for those nearing the end of life. In essence, hospice is a form of palliative care, but not all palliative care is hospice.

Benefits of Palliative Care

Palliative care offers a wide range of benefits for patients and their families, regardless of the stage of their illness:

- **Symptom Management:** Palliative care specialists are experts in managing pain, nausea, fatigue, shortness of breath, and other distressing symptoms associated with serious illness. Effective symptom control improves comfort and quality of life.

- **Improved Quality of Life:** By addressing physical, emotional, and psychosocial needs, palliative care enhances overall quality of life. Patients can experience greater comfort, reduced stress, and increased well-being.

- **Enhanced Communication:** Palliative care teams facilitate open and honest communication between patients, families, and healthcare providers. This helps ensure that everyone is informed and involved in decision-making.

- **Better Decision-Making:** Palliative care helps patients and families make informed decisions about their care, aligning treatment with their values and preferences. It empowers them to actively participate in their care planning.

- **Emotional and Psychosocial Support:** Palliative care addresses emotional distress, anxiety, depression, and other psychosocial challenges associated with serious illness. It provides counseling, support groups, and other resources to help patients and families cope.

- **Spiritual Support:** Palliative care recognizes the importance of spiritual well-being and offers support to patients and families exploring their spiritual needs and finding meaning and purpose in their experiences.

- **Reduced Hospitalizations and Emergency Room Visits:** By effectively managing symptoms and providing proactive care, palliative care can reduce the need for hospitalizations and emergency room visits, leading to a more comfortable and peaceful experience.

- **Improved Patient and Family Satisfaction:** Studies have shown that patients and families receiving palliative care report higher levels of satisfaction with their care.

Benefits of Hospice Care

Hospice care builds upon the principles of palliative care, offering comprehensive support to individuals nearing the end of life:

- **Comprehensive Care:** Hospice provides a holistic approach to care, addressing physical, emotional, social, and spiritual needs. It involves a team of professionals, including doctors, nurses, social workers, chaplains, and volunteers, working together to provide comprehensive support.

- **Focus on Comfort and Dignity:** Hospice prioritizes comfort and dignity, ensuring that patients are as comfortable as possible during their final days. It focuses on managing symptoms and providing emotional and spiritual support.

- **Pain Management:** Hospice experts are skilled in managing pain and other distressing symptoms, ensuring that patients are comfortable and can maintain their quality of life.

- **Emotional and Spiritual Support:** Hospice provides emotional and spiritual support to both patients and their families. Chaplains offer spiritual guidance and counseling, while social workers address emotional and psychosocial needs.

- **Family Support:** Hospice recognizes that the entire family is affected by the illness and provides support to caregivers and other family members. This includes education, counseling, respite care, and bereavement support.

- **Bereavement Services:** Hospice provides bereavement services to families for up to a year after the death of their loved one, helping them navigate the grieving process.

- **Respite Care:** Hospice offers respite care, providing temporary relief for caregivers, allowing them to take breaks and attend to their own needs.

- **Medical Equipment and Supplies:** Hospice provides all necessary medical equipment and supplies related to the terminal illness, reducing the burden on families.

- **Medication Management:** Hospice nurses manage medications, ensuring that patients receive the appropriate medications for symptom control.

- **24/7 Availability:** Hospice provides 24/7 availability, ensuring that patients and families have access to support whenever they need it.

Choosing Between Palliative Care and Hospice

The decision to pursue palliative care or hospice depends on the individual's specific circumstances, including their diagnosis, prognosis, and goals of care. Palliative care can be appropriate at any stage of a serious illness, while hospice is specifically for those nearing the end of life. It's important to discuss these options with your healthcare provider to determine the best approach for your situation.

Accessing Hospice and Palliative Care

- **Talk to Your Doctor:** Discuss your options with your physician. They can assess your needs and make recommendations for palliative care or hospice.

- **Contact a Hospice or Palliative Care Provider:** Many hospitals and healthcare systems have dedicated palliative care departments. You can also find hospice and palliative care providers in your community.

- **Check with Your Insurance Provider:** Most insurance plans, including Medicare and Medicaid, cover hospice and palliative care services. Contact your insurance provider to inquire about your coverage.

Overcoming Barriers to Access

Despite the numerous benefits, several barriers can prevent individuals from accessing hospice and palliative care:

- **Lack of Awareness:** Many people are not aware of the availability or benefits of these services.

- **Misconceptions:** Some people believe that hospice is only for those who are actively dying or that it means "giving up."

- **Physician Reluctance:** Some physicians may be hesitant to refer patients to hospice or palliative care.

- **Cultural Barriers:** Cultural beliefs and values can influence attitudes towards end-of-life care.

The Role of Caregivers in Promoting Access

Caregivers can play a vital role in promoting access to hospice and palliative care by:

- **Educating Themselves:** Learn about the benefits of these services and share this information with their loved ones and other family members.

- **Advocating for Their Loved One:** Talk to their loved one's physician about the possibility of hospice or palliative care.

- **Finding a Provider:** Research and identify hospice and palliative care providers in their community.

- **Addressing Concerns:** Address any misconceptions or concerns that their loved one or other family members may have about these services.

Eligibility Criteria for Hospice Care

To be eligible for hospice care, individuals must meet specific criteria:

- **Terminal Illness:** A physician must certify that the individual has a terminal illness with a life expectancy of six months or less, if the illness runs its normal course. This prognosis is based on the physician's clinical judgment and the natural progression of the disease.

- **Election of Hospice Benefit:** The individual must elect to receive hospice care and forgo curative treatment for the terminal illness. This signifies a shift in focus from attempting to cure the illness to prioritizing comfort and quality of life.

- **Willingness to Receive Palliative Care:** While hospice focuses on comfort rather than cure, it does not mean abandoning all medical care. Palliative care remains a core component of hospice, addressing symptoms and maximizing comfort.

Eligibility Criteria for Palliative Care

Palliative care has broader eligibility criteria than hospice care:

- **Serious Illness:** Individuals with any serious illness, regardless of stage or prognosis, are eligible for palliative care. This includes chronic conditions like cancer, heart failure, lung disease, dementia, and Parkinson's disease.

- **Focus on Quality of Life:** The primary focus is on improving quality of life by managing symptoms, addressing emotional and psychosocial needs, and supporting informed decision-making.

Accessing Hospice and Palliative Care

Accessing these services involves several steps:

1. **Talk to Your Doctor:** Discuss your concerns and explore options with your physician. They can assess your needs, make

recommendations, and provide referrals.

2. **Contact a Hospice or Palliative Care Provider:** Research and contact hospice and palliative care providers in your community. Many hospitals and healthcare systems have dedicated departments.

3. **Check with Your Insurance Provider:** Most insurance plans, including Medicare and Medicaid, cover hospice and palliative care services. Contact your provider to understand your coverage.

4. **Gather Necessary Documentation:** Be prepared to provide medical records and other relevant information to the hospice or palliative care provider.

5. **Schedule an Evaluation:** A nurse or other healthcare professional will conduct an evaluation to determine eligibility and develop a personalized care plan.

Overcoming Barriers to Access

Several factors can hinder access to hospice and palliative care:

- **Lack of Awareness:** Many individuals and families are unaware of the availability and benefits of these services.

- **Misconceptions:** Some believe hospice is only for the actively dying or that it means "giving up."

- **Physician Hesitancy:** Some physicians may be reluctant to refer patients to hospice or palliative care.

- **Cultural Barriers:** Cultural beliefs and values can influence attitudes towards end-of-life care.

The Role of Caregivers in Promoting Access

Caregivers are vital in advocating for their loved ones:

- **Educate Themselves:** Learn about the benefits of hospice and palliative care.

- **Discuss Options:** Talk to your loved one and other family members.

- **Advocate with Physicians:** Discuss these options with the physician.

- **Find a Provider:** Research and identify providers in your area.

- **Address Concerns:** Address any misconceptions or fears.

Financial Considerations

- **Medicare Hospice Benefit:** Medicare covers hospice care for eligible individuals.

- **Medicaid Coverage:** Medicaid also covers hospice and palliative care in many states.

- **Private Insurance:** Most private insurance plans offer coverage.

- **Financial Assistance:** Some organizations offer financial assistance for those who qualify.

Choosing a Hospice or Palliative Care Provider

Consider the following factors:

- **Accreditation and Certification:** Look for providers that are accredited

Chapter 19

Legal and Financial Considerations

Amidst the emotional weight of this experience, practical matters such as legal documents, financial management, and advance care planning can seem daunting. However, addressing these practicalities proactively is not only a responsible act but also a profound expression of love and care. It provides peace of mind for both the individual receiving care and their family, allowing them to focus on what truly matters: cherishing precious moments and ensuring a smooth transition.

The Importance of Practical Planning

Planning for end-of-life care involves more than just medical decisions. Addressing practical matters is equally important for ensuring a smooth and dignified transition. These practical considerations alleviate stress, prevent potential conflicts, and allow the individual to maintain control over their affairs to the greatest extent possible.

Key Practical Matters to Address

Wills and Estate Planning

- **The Role of a Will:** A will is a legal document that outlines how an individual's assets and property should be distributed after their death. It also designates an executor to manage the estate and can include provisions for guardianship of minor children. Having a valid will is crucial for ensuring that the individual's wishes are respected and that their loved ones are protected.

- **Creating or Updating a Will:** If a will does not exist, it's essential to create one. If a will exists, it should be reviewed and updated to reflect current wishes and circumstances. An attorney specializing in estate planning can provide guidance and ensure the will is legally sound.

- **Key Considerations in a Will:** These include:
  - Distribution of assets (real estate, bank accounts, investments, personal belongings)

  - Designation of an executor (responsible for managing the estate)

  - Guardianship of minor children (if applicable)

  - Charitable bequests (if desired)

  - Funeral arrangements (optional)

Power of Attorney (POA)

- **Types of Power of Attorney:** A Power of Attorney is a legal document that grants someone (the agent or attorney-in-fact) the authority to act on behalf of another person (the principal) in specific matters. There are different types of POAs:

  - **General POA:** Grants broad powers to the agent.

  - **Limited POA:** Grants specific powers for particular situations.

  - **Durable POA:** Remains in effect even if the principal becomes incapacitated.

  - **Healthcare POA:** Specifically grants authority to make healthcare decisions.

- **Importance of a Durable POA:** A durable POA is particularly important in end-of-life care, as it ensures that someone can manage the individual's financial and legal affairs if they become unable to do so themselves.

- **Choosing an Agent:** The agent should be someone trusted and capable, who understands the principal's wishes and is willing to act in their best interest.

Advance Directives

- **Purpose of Advance Directives:** Advance directives are legal documents that allow individuals to express their wishes regarding medical care if they become unable to communicate their decisions. They ensure that their preferences are respected and that their loved ones are not burdened with making difficult choices in a crisis.

- **Types of Advance Directives**

    o **Living Will:** Outlines specific medical treatments the individual wishes to receive or refuse in certain situations, such as life-sustaining measures.

    o **Healthcare Proxy (Durable Power of Attorney for Healthcare):** Designates a person (the proxy) to make healthcare decisions on the individual's behalf when they are unable to communicate.

- **Importance of Open Communication:** It's crucial to have open and honest conversations with family members and healthcare providers about advance directives to ensure everyone understands the individual's wishes.

Managing Finances

- **Organizing Financial Documents:** Gather all important financial documents, including bank statements, investment records, insurance policies, and tax returns, in one place. This will make it easier for the designated agent or executor to manage finances.

- **Paying Bills and Managing Accounts:** Ensure that someone is authorized to pay bills and manage financial accounts if the individual becomes incapacitated. This may involve setting up online banking access or granting access to a trusted family member.

- **Reviewing Insurance Policies:** Review life insurance policies, health insurance coverage, and other insurance policies to understand benefits and ensure they are up-to-date.

- **Planning for Funeral Expenses:** Discuss funeral arrangements and consider pre-planning or setting aside funds to cover these expenses.

Other Important Considerations

- **Digital Assets:** Consider managing digital assets, such as online accounts, social media profiles, and email accounts. Designate someone to manage or close these accounts after death.

- **Personal Belongings:** Discuss the distribution of personal belongings, such as family heirlooms, sentimental items, and other possessions. Creating a list or documenting wishes can prevent disputes among family members.

- **Pet Care:** Make arrangements for the care of pets if the individual is unable to provide care.

- **Communication with Healthcare Providers:** Maintain open communication with healthcare providers to ensure everyone is informed about the individual's wishes and care plan.

- **Support for Caregivers:** Recognize the emotional and practical needs of caregivers and ensure they have access to support resources.

Practical Tips for Addressing These Matters

- **Start Early:** Addressing these matters sooner rather than later allows for thoughtful planning and reduces stress during a crisis.

- **Seek Professional Guidance:** Consult with attorneys, financial advisors, and other professionals for expert advice and assistance.

- **Open Communication:** Have open and honest conversations with family members and loved ones about wishes and plans.

- **Document Everything:** Keep all important documents organized and easily accessible.

- **Regularly Review and Update:** Review and update wills, POAs, and advance directives periodically or as circumstances change.

- **Utilize Online Resources:** Numerous online resources offer information and guidance on end-of-life planning.

Resources for Assistance

- **National Hospice and Palliative Care Organization (NHPCO):** Provides resources on end-of-life care planning.

- **AARP:** Offers information and resources for seniors and their families, including guidance on legal and financial matters.

- **National Council on Aging (NCOA):** Provides resources on aging-related issues, including end-of-life planning.

- **Area Agencies on Aging (AAA):** Connect seniors and their caregivers with local resources, including legal and financial assistance.

- **Elder Law Attorneys:** Specialize in legal issues related to aging, including wills, POAs, and advance directives.

- **Financial Advisors:** Can provide guidance on financial planning and management.

Addressing practical matters during end-of-life care is an essential part of ensuring a smooth and dignified transition. By proactively planning for legal, financial, and personal affairs, individuals can maintain control over their lives to the greatest extent possible and provide peace of mind for themselves and their loved ones. While these conversations may be difficult, they are an act of love and responsibility, allowing families to focus on what truly matters: cherishing precious moments and providing compassionate care during a time of profound transition. By utilizing available resources and seeking professional guidance, caregivers can navigate these practicalities with greater confidence and ensure that their loved one's wishes are respected and their legacy is preserved.

Chapter 20

Resources and Support Organizations

National Organizations

- **AARP (American Association of Retired Persons):** (aarp.org) Offers a wide range of resources for seniors and their caregivers, including articles, guides, and a caregiver resource center.

- **ARCH National Respite Network and Resource Center:** (archrespite.org) Provides information and resources on respite care, including a national respite locator.

- **Caregiver Action Network (CAN):** (caregiveraction.org) Offers support, education, and advocacy for family caregivers.

- **Family Caregiver Alliance (FCA):** (caregiver.org) Provides information, resources, and support for family caregivers, including state-specific resources.

- **HelpGuide.org:** (helpguide.org) Offers comprehensive articles on caregiving, grief, and other related topics.

- **The National Alliance for Grieving Children:** (childrengrieve.org) Offers resources specifically for children and teens experiencing grief.

- **The Dougy Center:** (dougy.org) Provides support groups and resources for children, teens, young adults, and their families grieving a death.

- **The Compassionate Friends:** (compassionatefriends.org) Offers peer support groups for parents who have lost a child.

- **The Tragedy Assistance Program for Survivors (TAPS):** (taps.org) Provides support and resources for those grieving the loss of a military loved one.

- **The National Hospice and Palliative Care Organization (NHPCO):** (nhpco.org) Offers resources on hospice and palliative care, grief, and bereavement.

- **The Center for Loss and Life Transition:** (centerforloss.com) Provides resources, books, and workshops on grief and loss.

- **National Council on Aging (NCOA):** (ncoa.org) Offers resources on aging-related issues, including caregiving and end-of-life planning.

- **Alzheimer's Association:** (alz.org) Provides support and resources for individuals and families affected by Alzheimer's disease.

- **American Cancer Society:** (cancer.org) Offers support and resources for individuals and families facing cancer.

- **National Parkinson Foundation:** (parkinson.org) Offers support and resources for individuals and families affected by Parkinson's disease.

Local and Regional Resources

- **Your Local Area Agency on Aging (AAA):** This is often the best starting point. AAAs connect seniors and their caregivers with local resources, including respite care, home care, transportation, meals on wheels, and other support services. You can typically find your local AAA by searching online for "[your county/city] Area Agency on Aging."

- **Your State's Department of Aging or Human Services:** These agencies often have programs and resources related to caregiving and senior services.

- **Hospice and Palliative Care Organizations:** These organizations provide end-of-life care and often offer bereavement services to families and the community.

- **Hospitals and Healthcare Systems:** Many hospitals have social work departments that can assist with finding community resources, including caregiver support groups and respite care options.

- **Senior Centers:** Local senior centers often provide information about respite options and may even offer some respite services themselves, such as adult day care.

- **Mental Health Professionals:** Therapists and counselors specializing in grief and loss can provide individual or family therapy.

- **Places of Worship:** Many religious communities offer grief support groups or individual counseling through their clergy or lay leaders.

- **Community Centers:** Some community centers offer grief support groups or workshops.

- **Disability-Specific Organizations:** If your loved one has a specific disability (e.g., Alzheimer's, Parkinson's), organizations related to that condition may have caregiver support resources.

Online Search Strategies

- **Search for "caregiver support [your city/state]" or "end-of-life care resources [your city/state]":** This will help you find local resources.

- **Look for "[disease name] caregiver support groups"**: This can connect you with groups specific to your loved one's condition.

Tips for Finding the Right Resources

- **Consider your specific needs:** Are you looking for respite care, emotional support, financial assistance, or help with legal matters?

- **Think about your loved one's needs:** What kind of care does your loved one require?

- **Explore different options:** Don't be afraid to try different resources until you find what works best for you and your family.

- **Don't hesitate to ask for help:** Many caregivers hesitate to seek help, but it's important to remember that you don't have to do this alone.

Utilizing available resources can make a significant difference in your ability to provide compassionate care while also taking care of yourself.

Chapter 21

Checklist for End-of-Life Planning

Checklist for Organized and Effective Care

Caregiving, particularly during end-of-life situations, can feel like navigating uncharted waters. Amidst the emotional weight and complex medical decisions, the sheer volume of practical tasks can be overwhelming. This chapter offers a comprehensive checklist designed to help caregivers organize and manage essential tasks, empowering them to provide the best possible care while also preserving their own well-being. This "Caregiver's Compass" is not meant to be exhaustive, as each caregiving situation is unique, but it provides a framework for staying organized and focused on what matters most.

Initial Assessment and Information Gathering

- [ ] **Loved One's Information:** Full name, date of birth, Social Security number, insurance information (Medicare, Medicaid, private insurance), physician contact information, allergies, medical history.

- [ ] **Caregiver Information:** Contact information for primary caregiver(s), including emergency contacts.

- [ ] **Legal Documents:** Location of will, power of attorney (POA), advance directives (living will, healthcare proxy), and any other relevant legal documents.

- [ ] **Financial Information:** Location of bank accounts, investment records, insurance policies, and other financial documents.

- [ ] **Medical Information:** List of current medications (name, dosage, frequency), medical conditions, past surgeries, and immunizations.

- [ ] **Support Network:** Contact information for family members, friends, or other individuals who can provide support.

Medical Management

- [ ] **Physician Appointments:** Schedule and keep track of all medical appointments. Prepare questions in advance.

- [ ] **Medication Management:** Create a medication schedule and ensure medications are taken as prescribed. Refill prescriptions on time. Monitor for side effects.

- [ ] **Symptom Tracking:** Keep a record of symptoms, including frequency, severity, and any triggers. Communicate this information to the medical team.

- [ ] **Medical Equipment:** Arrange for necessary medical equipment (e.g., hospital bed, oxygen, walker) and ensure proper usage.

- [ ] **Emergency Plan:** Develop an emergency plan, including contact information for emergency services and instructions for specific situations.

- [ ] **Communication with Medical Team:** Maintain regular communication with doctors, nurses, and other healthcare providers. Document all communication.

Personal Care

- [ ] **Daily Routine:** Establish a daily routine that includes bathing, dressing, grooming, and meals.

- [ ] **Hygiene:** Ensure proper hygiene, including oral care, skin care, and nail care.

- [ ] **Nutrition:** Plan and prepare nutritious meals, considering any dietary restrictions or preferences.

- [ ] **Mobility:** Assist with mobility as needed, including walking, transfers, and exercise.

- [ ] **Comfort:** Ensure the loved one's comfort, including appropriate clothing, positioning, and temperature.

Financial and Legal Matters

- [ ] **Financial Management:** Manage finances, including paying bills, managing bank accounts, and handling insurance claims.

- [ ] **Legal Documents:** Ensure all legal documents are in order and easily accessible.

- [ ] **Advance Care Planning:** Discuss and document end-of-life wishes, including preferences for medical treatment and care.

- [ ] **Estate Planning:** Review and update estate plans, including wills and beneficiary designations.

Emotional and Social Support

- [ ] **Emotional Support:** Provide emotional support, including listening, offering comfort, and validating feelings.

- [ ] **Social Activities:** Encourage social interaction and engagement in activities that bring joy.

- [ ] **Respite Care:** Arrange for respite care to allow for breaks and self-care.

- [ ] **Support Groups:** Connect with support groups for caregivers and individuals facing similar situations.

- [ ] **Mental Health:** Prioritize mental health and seek professional help if needed.

Home Environment

- [ ] **Safety:** Ensure a safe home environment, including removing hazards and installing safety equipment.

- [ ] **Accessibility:** Make necessary modifications to improve accessibility, such as ramps, grab bars, and widened doorways.

- [ ] **Cleanliness:** Maintain a clean and organized home environment.

- [ ] **Comfort:** Create a comfortable and relaxing atmosphere.

End-of-Life Planning (If Applicable)

- [ ] **Hospice Care:** Explore hospice care options and eligibility requirements.

- [ ] **Funeral Arrangements:** Discuss and document funeral arrangements, including preferences for burial or cremation.

- [ ] **Memorial Plans:** Plan a memorial service or other way to honor the loved one's memory.

- [ ] **Bereavement Support:** Identify bereavement support resources for family members.

Caregiver Well-being

- [ ] **Self-Care:** Prioritize self-care, including healthy eating, exercise, and adequate sleep.

- [ ] **Stress Management:** Practice stress management techniques, such as mindfulness, meditation, or deep breathing exercises.

- [ ] **Boundaries:** Set boundaries and say no to additional responsibilities when needed.

- [ ] **Support System:** Build a strong support system of family, friends, or other caregivers.

- [ ] **Professional Help:** Seek professional help if needed, including therapy or counseling.

Ongoing Tasks and Reminders

- [ ] **Regularly Review and Update:** Review and update this checklist regularly as needs change.

- [ ] **Prioritize Tasks:** Prioritize tasks based on urgency and importance.

- [ ] **Delegate Tasks:** Delegate tasks to other family members or friends when possible.

- [ ] **Seek Assistance:** Don't hesitate to ask for help from professionals, volunteers, or community resources.

Using this Checklist

This Caregiver's Compass is a dynamic tool. Regularly review and update it to ensure it continues to meet your evolving needs. Remember, you are not alone in this journey. Utilize this checklist as a guide, seek support when needed, and prioritize both the care of your loved one and your own well-being.

Chapter 22

Setting the Stage for Transition

Creating a peaceful and supportive environment for a loved one's passing is a deeply personal and meaningful act of caregiving. It's about fostering comfort, dignity, and a sense of connection during this sacred time. When staging the environment, focus on both physical and emotional aspects.

Physical Environment

- **Comfort is Key**

    - ○ **Bedding:** Use soft, comfortable sheets and blankets. Consider a specialized mattress or topper if needed to prevent pressure sores and enhance comfort. Adjust pillows for optimal support.

    - ○ **Temperature:** Maintain a comfortable room temperature. Too hot or too cold can add to discomfort. Ask your loved one for their preference if possible.

    - ○ **Lighting:** Soft, warm lighting is generally preferred. Avoid harsh overhead lights. Consider lamps with adjustable settings. Natural light can be soothing, but be mindful of glare.

- o **Noise:** Minimize noise from televisions, radios, or conversations. Soft, calming music or nature sounds may be welcome. Respect silence if preferred.

- o **Air Quality:** Ensure good ventilation and fresh air. Avoid strong scents or perfumes that might be irritating. Aromatherapy with calming essential oils (like lavender or chamomile, if tolerated) can be considered, but proceed cautiously and consult with medical professionals if needed.

- o **Cleanliness:** Maintain a clean and tidy room. Fresh linens and a clutter-free space can contribute to a sense of peace.

- **Accessibility and Safety**

  - o **Easy Access:** Ensure easy access to the bed, bathroom, and other frequently used areas. Remove any tripping hazards.

  - o **Safety Measures:** Install grab bars in the bathroom if needed. Keep the call bell within easy reach.

- Medication and Supplies: Keep medications and necessary medical supplies readily accessible but safely stored.

- **Personal Touches**

  - **Familiar Objects:** Place familiar and comforting objects nearby, such as photos, artwork, religious items, or favorite books. These can provide a sense of connection and comfort.

  - **Meaningful Items:** Include items that hold special meaning for your loved one. This could be a cherished blanket, a piece of jewelry, or a letter from a loved one.

  - **Nature:** If possible, bring in elements of nature, such as flowers or a small plant. A view of nature through a window can also be calming.

Emotional and Spiritual Environment

- **Presence and Connection**

  - **Be Present:** Your presence is the most valuable gift you can offer. Simply being there, holding a hand, and offering quiet companionship can provide immense comfort.

- ○ **Active Listening:** Listen attentively to your loved one's thoughts and feelings, even if they are expressed nonverbally.

- ○ **Respectful Communication:** Communicate with respect, honesty, and compassion. Speak calmly and gently.

- ○ **Emotional Support:** Offer emotional support and reassurance. Let your loved one know that they are loved and not alone.

- **Spiritual Considerations**

  - ○ **Respect Beliefs:** Respect your loved one's spiritual beliefs and practices.

  - ○ **Spiritual Support:** If desired, facilitate visits from clergy, spiritual advisors, or other spiritual support figures.

  - ○ **Sacred Space:** Create a small sacred space in the room if appropriate, with religious items or other meaningful symbols.

- **Creating a Peaceful Atmosphere**

- o **Music:** Play soft, calming music or nature sounds if desired. Choose music that has special meaning or evokes positive memories.

- o **Silence:** Respect the need for silence if your loved one prefers it.

- o **Rituals:** If appropriate, engage in meaningful rituals, such as prayer, meditation, or reading scriptures.

- **Family and Friends**

  - o **Visits:** Encourage visits from close family members and friends, if your loved one is receptive. Coordinate visits to avoid overwhelming the individual.

  - o **Shared Memories:** Share stories and memories with your loved one. This can be a way to celebrate their life and provide comfort.

Practical Considerations

- **Medical Equipment:** If medical equipment is needed, ensure it is placed discreetly and does not interfere with the overall peaceful atmosphere.

- **Caregiver Comfort:** Consider the comfort of caregivers as well. Have a comfortable chair nearby and ensure access to refreshments and bathroom facilities.

- **Privacy:** Respect the need for privacy for both the individual and their loved ones.

Important Reminders

- **Individual Preferences:** The most important thing is to tailor the environment to your loved one's individual preferences and needs.

- **Flexibility:** Be flexible and adaptable. Needs and preferences may change as the dying process progresses.

- **Focus on Comfort:** The primary goal is to create a comfortable, peaceful, and supportive environment that promotes dignity and connection.

Living Funeral

Hosting a living funeral, also known as a celebration of life, a life review, or a pre-funeral gathering, can be a beautiful and meaningful way to honor a loved one while they are still present. It allows them to hear tributes, share stories, and connect with those they cherish before they pass.

Benefits for the Person Passing

- **Opportunity to Receive Love and Appreciation:** A living funeral allows the individual to hear firsthand how they have impacted the lives of others. They can receive expressions of love, gratitude, and admiration from family and friends, which can be incredibly comforting and affirming.

- **Sense of Completion and Closure:** It provides a chance to say goodbye and express any unfinished business. They can share their love, wisdom, and final wishes with loved ones, fostering a sense of peace and completion.

- **Control and Agency:** In a situation where much may feel out of control, a living funeral allows the individual to actively participate in planning and shaping their own memorial. This can provide a sense of agency and empowerment.

- **Celebration of Life:** It shifts the focus from death to celebrating a life well-lived. This can be a powerful and positive experience, reminding them of the joy and love they have shared.

- **Reduced Anxiety and Fear:** By addressing end-of-life matters openly and surrounded by loved ones, a living funeral can help reduce anxiety and fear about death.

- **Strengthened Bonds:** It provides an opportunity for deep connection and meaningful conversations with family and friends, strengthening bonds during a precious time.

- **Leave a Legacy:** A living funeral can be a way to leave a lasting legacy. They can share their stories, values, and life lessons with future generations.

Benefits for the Family

- **Opportunity to Express Love and Gratitude:** Family members can express their love, appreciation, and gratitude to the individual while they are still present. This can be a powerful and healing experience.

- **Shared Grief and Support:** A living funeral provides a space for family and friends to gather, share their grief, and offer support to one another. This can be particularly helpful for those who are struggling with anticipatory grief.

- **Memories and Stories:** It creates an opportunity to share stories and memories, celebrating the individual's life and legacy. These shared memories can be a source of comfort and strength in the future.

- **Closure and Healing:** Saying goodbye in a meaningful way can help family members begin the grieving process and find closure. It can reduce feelings of regret or unfinished business.

- **Strengthened Family Bonds:** Planning and participating in a living funeral can bring families closer together, creating a shared experience of love and support.

- **Honoring Wishes:** It allows the family to honor the wishes of their loved one and ensure that their life is celebrated in a way that is meaningful to them.

- **Preparation for Loss:** While not replacing the grieving process after death, a living funeral can help family members prepare for the loss and begin to adjust to the idea of life without their loved one.

- **Lasting Memories:** The living funeral creates lasting memories that family members can cherish in the years to come. These memories can be a source of comfort and strength during difficult times.

Hosting the Event

Discuss it with your loved one

- **Their Wishes:** This is paramount. A living funeral is for them, so their comfort and preferences should guide every decision. Discuss the idea openly and respectfully. If they're not comfortable with a formal event, explore alternative ways to celebrate their life.

- **Their Vision:** What kind of gathering do they envision? Formal or informal? Large or small? Do they have specific requests for music, readings, or activities?

- **Timing:** When would they like to hold the gathering? Consider their energy levels and overall health.

Planning the Logistics

- **Date and Time:** Choose a date and time that works well for your loved one and key family members and friends. Be mindful of their energy levels and any medical appointments.

- **Location:** Select a location that is accessible and comfortable. This could be their home, a community center, a park, a church, or even a restaurant. Consider the size of the gathering and the overall atmosphere you want to create.

- **Guest List:** Work with your loved one to create a guest list of important people in their lives. Consider sending invitations well in advance.

- **Invitations:** Design invitations that reflect the tone of the gathering. Include information about the date, time, location, and any special instructions (e.g., dress code, contributions).

- **Food and Drinks:** Plan for food and drinks. This could range from a simple buffet to a more formal meal. Consider your loved one's preferences and dietary needs.

- **Decorations:** Create a warm and inviting atmosphere with decorations that reflect your loved one's personality and interests. This could include photos, artwork, flowers, or other meaningful items.

- **Program or Activities:** Plan a program or activities that will honor your loved one's life. This could include:
  - Sharing stories and memories
  - Reading poems or favorite passages
  - Playing music
  - Showing photos or videos
  - Open mic for guests to share tributes
  - A symbolic act (e.g., planting a tree, releasing balloons)

- **Music:** Choose music that has special meaning for your loved one or that creates the desired atmosphere.

- **Photography/Videography:** Consider hiring a photographer or videographer to capture the event. This can create lasting memories for family and friends.

- **Tributes and Speeches:** Encourage guests to prepare short tributes or speeches to share during the gathering.

- **Memory Book or Guest Book:** Provide a memory book or guest book for guests to write messages and share their condolences.

During the Living Funeral

- **Welcome Guests:** Designate someone to welcome guests and make them feel comfortable.

- **Facilitate the Program:** Have someone act as the emcee or facilitator to guide the program and ensure that everything runs smoothly.

- **Encourage Participation:** Create opportunities for guests to participate, such as sharing stories, reading tributes, or offering words of support.

- **Keep it Focused and Positive:** While acknowledging the sadness of the situation, focus on celebrating the loved one's life and the positive impact they have had on others.

- **Be Flexible:** Be prepared to adapt the program as needed. The most important thing is to create a meaningful and memorable experience for your loved one and their guests.

- **Capture the Moments:** Take photos and videos to document the event and create lasting memories.

After the Living Funeral

- **Thank You Notes:** Send thank you notes to guests for their attendance and contributions.

- **Reflect and Cherish:** Take time to reflect on the event and cherish the memories created.

- **Continue Support:** Offer ongoing support to your loved one and other family members and friends.

Important Considerations

- **Emotional Sensitivity:** Be mindful of the emotional needs of everyone involved. Grief is a complex and personal process, and some guests may be experiencing a range of emotions.

- **Respectful Atmosphere:** Create a respectful and supportive atmosphere where everyone feels comfortable sharing their thoughts and feelings.

- **Focus on Celebration:** While acknowledging the impending loss, the primary focus should be on celebrating the loved one's life and the positive impact they have had on others.

- **Professional Help:** Consider involving a professional, such as a celebrant or a grief counselor, to help plan and facilitate the living funeral.

Hosting a living funeral can be a profound and healing experience for everyone involved. It provides an opportunity to express love, gratitude, and appreciation while your loved one is still present, creating lasting memories and offering comfort during a difficult time. By carefully planning and paying attention to the details, you can create a beautiful and

meaningful tribute that honors your loved one's life
and legacy.

Chapter 23

Caregivers Guilt

Understanding and Releasing Caregiver Guilt

The death of a loved one after a period of caregiving often brings a complex mix of emotions. Among these, guilt can be particularly pervasive and difficult to navigate. Caregiver guilt isn't simply regret; it's a tangled web of "what ifs," self-blame, and a deep sense of responsibility that can linger long after the funeral. This chapter explores the multifaceted nature of caregiver guilt, examining its common roots, offering strategies for understanding and processing it, and ultimately, guiding you towards self-compassion and healing.

The Weight of "What Ifs": Unpacking the Roots of Guilt

Caregiver guilt stems from a variety of sources, often intertwined and deeply personal. Understanding these roots is the first step toward untangling the web and finding a path toward peace.

- **"I Didn't Do Enough":** This is a common refrain, particularly for those who provided extensive care. Caregivers often question whether they could have done more, tried harder, or made different choices. Even when care was exceptional, the feeling of inadequacy can persist.

- **Second-Guessing Decisions:** End-of-life care often involves difficult medical decisions. Caregivers may second-guess choices made about treatment, pain management, or end-of-life interventions, wondering if a different path would have led to a different outcome.

- **Regret Over Missed Opportunities:** Caregiving can be all-consuming, sometimes leaving little time for other things. Caregivers may feel guilty about missed opportunities – missed vacations, neglected friendships, or simply not spending enough quality time outside of caregiving duties.

- **Unresolved Relationship Issues:** If there were unresolved conflicts or strained relationships with the loved one, these issues can fuel guilt. Caregivers may regret not having the chance to mend fences or say what needed to be said.

- **Feeling Relief After a Long Illness:** Paradoxically, feeling relief after a prolonged and challenging illness can also trigger guilt. Caregivers may question the appropriateness of feeling relieved, fearing it implies a lack of love or grief.

- **Societal Expectations and Unrealistic Standards:** Society often portrays caregivers as selfless saints, setting an impossibly high bar. Caregivers may feel guilty for not living up to these unrealistic expectations, for needing breaks, or for experiencing negative emotions.

- **The Burden of Responsibility:** Caregivers often carry a heavy burden of responsibility, feeling solely accountable for their loved one's well-being. This sense of responsibility can morph into guilt, especially when the outcome is beyond anyone's control.

The Many Faces of Guilt: Recognizing its Manifestations

Guilt can manifest in various ways, impacting not only emotional well-being but also physical and mental health. Recognizing these manifestations is crucial for addressing them effectively.

- **Emotional Turmoil:** Persistent feelings of sadness, regret, remorse, shame, and self-blame. These emotions can be intense and overwhelming, impacting daily life.

- **Physical Symptoms:** Guilt can manifest physically through fatigue, sleep disturbances, changes in appetite, headaches, and other stress-related ailments.

- **Cognitive Difficulties:** Difficulty concentrating, memory problems, and intrusive thoughts related to caregiving experiences.

- **Behavioral Changes:** Social withdrawal, irritability, anxiety, and even substance abuse can be linked to unresolved guilt.

Untangling the Web: Strategies for Processing Guilt

Processing caregiver guilt is a journey, not a destination. It requires self-compassion, patience, and a willingness to confront difficult emotions. The following strategies can help:

- **Acknowledge and Validate Your Feelings:** The first step is to acknowledge the guilt without judgment. Recognize that these feelings are normal, especially given the challenging circumstances of caregiving. Don't try to suppress or minimize your emotions.

- **Challenge Negative Thoughts:** Guilt often stems from negative and often distorted thinking. Challenge these thoughts by asking yourself: "Is this thought realistic?" "What evidence supports this thought?" "Is there another way to look at this situation?"

- **Reframe Your Perspective:** Try to view your caregiving experience with compassion. Recognize that you did the best you could with the resources and knowledge you had at the time. Focus on the love and dedication you demonstrated.

- **Remember the Positive Moments:** Counter negative thoughts by focusing on the positive aspects of your caregiving experience. Recall the moments of connection, the expressions of gratitude, and the ways you made your loved one's life better.

- **Separate What You Could Control from What You Couldn't:** It's crucial to distinguish between what was within your control and what was not. You could control your actions, your love, and your dedication, but you couldn't control the course of the illness or the ultimate outcome.

- **Forgive Yourself:** Forgiveness is a crucial step in healing. It doesn't mean condoning any mistakes you might have made, but it does mean releasing yourself from the burden of guilt. Practice self-compassion and offer yourself the same forgiveness you would offer a friend in a similar situation.

- **Seek Support:** Talking about your feelings with trusted friends, family members, or a therapist can be incredibly helpful. Sharing your experience with others who understand can provide validation and support.

- **Join a Support Group:** Connecting with other caregivers who have experienced similar losses can be particularly valuable. Support groups offer a safe space to share experiences, learn coping strategies, and realize you are not alone.

- **Professional Counseling:** If guilt is overwhelming or interfering with your daily life, consider seeking professional help from a therapist or counselor specializing in grief and loss. A therapist can provide guidance and support as you navigate the complexities of guilt and grief.

- **Focus on Self-Care:** Prioritize your physical and emotional well-being. Engage in activities that bring you joy, practice relaxation techniques, and ensure you are getting enough rest. Self-care is not selfish; it's essential for healing.

- **Honor Your Loved One's Memory:** Finding meaningful ways to honor your loved one's memory can be a powerful way to channel grief and guilt into something positive. This might involve creating a memorial, donating to a charity in their name, or carrying on a tradition they cherished.

The Journey Toward Healing

Healing from caregiver guilt is a process, not an event. There will be good days and bad days. Be patient with yourself, allow yourself to grieve, and remember that you are not alone. The love and care you provided made a difference, and that is something to be proud of. By practicing self-compassion, seeking support, and focusing on the positive aspects of your caregiving experience, you can release the burden of guilt and find peace in honoring your loved one's memory.

Chapter 24

Honoring Your Loved One

Creative Ways to Honor Your Loved One After They Pass

The death of a loved one leaves an irreplaceable void, a silence where laughter once echoed, and an emptiness where their presence once filled the room. Grief, a complex and deeply personal journey, intertwines with the desire to keep their memory alive, to honor their life, and to ensure their spirit continues to influence the world. While traditional memorials offer comfort, many seek more creative and personalized ways to celebrate their loved one's unique essence. There are a multitude of creative avenues for honoring your loved one after they pass, offering inspiration and practical ideas to keep their spirit alive for generations to come.

Celebrating Life, Not Just Mourning Death

The focus after a loss often centers on mourning, which is natural and necessary. However, equally important is celebrating the life lived, the joy shared, and the impact made. Shifting the narrative, even partially, towards celebration can be a powerful way to honor their memory.

Storytelling and Legacy:

1. **Oral Histories:** Gather family and friends to share stories and anecdotes about your loved one. Record these conversations to create an oral history, a precious keepsake for future generations.

2. **Written Tributes:** Encourage family and friends to write down their favorite memories or what they learned from your loved one. Compile these tributes into a book, a website, or a beautifully designed memory journal.

3. **Family Recipes:** If they had cherished family recipes, create a family cookbook in their honor. Share the recipes and the stories behind them, keeping their culinary legacy alive.

4. **Life Story Video:** Create a video montage of photos, videos, and music that tells the story of their life. Include interviews with family and friends sharing their favorite memories.

5. **Personalized Children's Book:** If they had a special connection with children, consider creating a children's book based on a story they used to tell, a lesson they taught, or a character inspired by them.

Acts of Kindness and Service

1. **Memorial Scholarship:** Establish a scholarship fund in their name to support

students pursuing education in a field they were passionate about.

2. **Charitable Donations:** Donate to a charity or cause they supported during their lifetime or one that reflects their values.

3. **Acts of Kindness Challenge:** Organize an "Acts of Kindness" challenge in their name, encouraging others to perform small acts of kindness in their community.

4. **Volunteer Work:** Volunteer your time to an organization they cared about. This could be anything from a local soup kitchen to an animal shelter.

Creative and Artistic Expressions

1. **Memorial Art Project:** Create a piece of art in their memory. This could be a painting, sculpture, quilt, or any other form of artistic expression.

2. **Personalized Music Playlist:** Compile a playlist of their favorite songs or music that reminds you of them. Share this playlist with family and friends.

3. **Poetry or Writing:** Write a poem, song, or short story that captures the essence of their life or your relationship with them.

4. **Memory Garden:** Plant a memorial garden with their favorite flowers or plants. Include a

personalized plaque or stone.

5. **Commissioned Artwork:** Commission a portrait, sculpture, or other piece of art that reflects their personality or a special memory.

Lasting Memorials and Physical Tributes

While digital and experiential tributes are powerful, physical memorials can provide a tangible connection to the past.

Personalized Memorials:

1. **Custom Headstone or Plaque:** Design a headstone or memorial plaque that reflects their personality, interests, or beliefs.

2. **Memorial Bench:** Place a memorial bench in a park, garden, or other location that was special to them.

3. **Cremation Jewelry:** Consider cremation jewelry, which allows you to keep a small portion of their ashes in a beautiful pendant or other piece of jewelry.

4. **Tattoo Memorial:** Some individuals choose to get a tattoo incorporating their loved one's initials, a significant symbol, or a meaningful quote.

Incorporating Ashes

1. **Scattering Ashes:** Scattering ashes in a meaningful location can be a powerful and cathartic experience.

2. **Ashes in Artwork:** Some companies specialize in incorporating ashes into artwork, such as paintings, sculptures, or even blown glass.

3. **Planting a Memorial Tree:** Certain companies offer services where ashes are mixed with soil and used to plant a memorial tree.

Keeping Their Spirit Alive in Daily Life

The most enduring tribute is often how we choose to live our own lives after the loss.

Living Their Values

Carry on Traditions: Continue family traditions or create new ones in their memory.

Embrace Their Passions: Pursue hobbies or interests they enjoyed.

Live with Intention: Strive to live your life in a way that reflects their values and the lessons they taught you.

Connecting with Nature

Visit Special Places: Visit places that were special to them or that they always wanted to visit.

Spend Time in Nature: Spend time in nature, reflecting on their life and the beauty of the world around you.

Acts of Remembrance

Anniversary or Birthday Celebrations: Celebrate their birthday or anniversary with a special meal, gathering, or act of remembrance.

Light a Candle: Light a candle in their memory on special occasions or during times of reflection.

Share Stories Regularly: Keep their memory alive by sharing stories and anecdotes with family and friends.

Honoring a loved one after they pass is a lifelong journey. It's about keeping their memory alive, celebrating their life, and finding ways to integrate their love and influence into your own life. There's no single "right" way to do this. Choose the methods that resonate most with you and allow you to express your love and grief in a way that feels authentic and meaningful. The most important thing is to keep their spirit alive in your heart and in your actions. Their legacy continues through you.

And so, we reach the end of this journey, a journey we've shared through these pages. "The Long Goodbye" is not a story with a neatly tied bow, nor a guidebook with all the answers. It is, instead, a testament to the messy, beautiful, and profoundly human experience of caring for a loved one as they approach the end of their life.

We've explored the challenges, the triumphs, the moments of heart-wrenching sorrow and unexpected joy. We've talked about the practicalities of caregiving, the legal and financial necessities, and the importance of advance care planning. We've delved into the emotional landscape, acknowledging the grief, the guilt, and the overwhelming love that often accompanies this phase of life.

If there's one thing I hope you take away from this book, it's that you are not alone. The feelings you experience—the exhaustion, the frustration, the unwavering devotion—are shared by countless others who have walked this path before you. And while the journey is undoubtedly difficult, it is also a sacred privilege.

Remember to be kind to yourself. Caregiving is a marathon, not a sprint. Allow yourself moments of respite, seek support from your network, and don't hesitate to ask for professional help when needed. Your well-being is essential, not only for your own sake but also for the sake of the person you are caring for.

As you navigate the complexities of end-of-life care, remember to cherish the moments. Embrace the opportunities for connection, for sharing stories, and for expressing your love. These moments, however fleeting, will become the precious memories you hold dear long after your loved one has passed.

The long goodbye is a process of letting go, but it is also a process of holding onto the love, the memories, and the enduring bond that will forever connect you. May you find strength, comfort, and peace as you walk this final chapter together. And may the lessons learned during this time enrich your life in ways you never imagined.

Made in the USA
Columbia, SC
13 March 2025

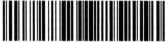

55054206R00226